# Medicine
## and the
# Management
## of Living

# Medicine and

*William Ray Arney & Bernard J. Bergen*

# the Management of Living

## Taming the Last Great Beast

The University of Chicago Press
Chicago and London

William Ray Arney is a Member of the Faculty at The
Evergreen State College (Olympia, Washington) and the
author of *Power and the Profession of Obstetrics,*
published by the University of Chicago Press in 1982.
Bernard J. Bergen is Adjunct Professor of Sociology at
Dartmouth College and Professor of Psychiatry at
Dartmouth Medical School. He is coauthor of *The Cold
Fire: Alienation and the Myth of Culture* (1976) and
coeditor of *Issues and Problems in Social Psychology*
(1965).

THE UNIVERSITY OF CHICAGO PRESS, CHICAGO 60637
THE UNIVERSITY OF CHICAGO PRESS, LTD., LONDON

93 92 91 90 89 88 87 86 85 84    5 4 3 2 1

*Library of Congress Cataloging in Publication Data*

Arney, William Ray.
   Medicine and the management of living.

   Includes index.
   1. Physician and patient.   2. Power (Social sciences)
3. Social medicine.   I. Bergen, Bernard J.   II. Title.
[DNLM: 1. Physician-patient relations.   2. Sociology,
Medical.   W 62 A748m]
R727.3.A76   1984        362.1'042        83-24380
ISBN 0-226-02792-9

To our students, who suffered us and whom we suffered as each tried to introduce a little disharmony into the others' lives

# Contents

# Acknowledgments

It is redundant to begin a book that is itself a preface with a preface. Nothing at all would have happened, however, without the support and valuable suggestions of others along the way. Eileen Crane conducted some of the research on teenage pregnancy. David Armstrong, Charles Bosk, Elise Boulding, Kenneth Boulding, Barbara Ehrenreich, Bruce Finnie, Michel Foucault, Stan Rosenberg, and Robert A. Scott read drafts of the manuscript and knew unerringly what was wrong. If it is still wrong, it is no fault of theirs. Thanks, finally, to the NAD for a fruitful party.

After this I saw in the night visions, and behold a fourth great beast, dreadful and terrible, and strong exceedingly; and it had great iron teeth: it devoured and brake in pieces, and stamped the residue with the feet of it: and it was diverse from all the beasts that were before it.

The Book of Daniel 7: 7

No one can conceive the variety of feelings which bore me onwards, like a hurricane, in the first enthusiasm of success. Life and death appeared to me ideal bounds, which I should first break through, and pour a torrent of light into our dark world. A new species would bless me as its creator and source; many happy and excellent natures would owe their being to me.

Frankenstein or The Modern Prometheus, 1818

# One

# Introduction

WE WISH TO INTERPRET an experience intimately familiar to almost everyone: the encounter between patients and physicians. The terms on which patients and physicians meet are changing in profound ways. The manner in which the cardinal elements of the medical encounter—the patient, the physician and the disease—relate to one another is changing.

To begin our interpretation of the modern medical encounter we should start not in the doctor's office but in the modern bookstore. A cursory glance at the shelves of bookstores today shows that we live in an age where people need to talk about the self. Books speak less and less about the facts of the world or the intimate experiences of others and more and more about how to make the self transparent. We read in order to find out how to express ourselves, how to assert ourselves, how to communicate and connect. It seems there is no experience, from birth to death, love to hate, suffering to joy that is privileged. We can learn how to express everything. Nothing need be held back or kept private. We call it an age of liberation.

Nowhere is this phenomenon more impressive than among those who have become medical patients. When the self begins to speak about its experience of suffering an illness, it confronts a rule that we all learned governed the traditional medical encounter: "You shall speak only about things the physician designates important to the medical encounter; otherwise, keep silent." When the self speaks of the experience of being or becoming a patient, it speaks about what is important to it, not necessarily about what is important to the physician. And there lies a potential conflict. Indeed, the modern bookstore suggests that patients, ex-patients and would-be patients are forming themselves into a social movement that is not unlike a rebellion. It seems that the self is asserting itself against medical indifference to the experiences and emotions that make up life, and it seems that the self is calling into question the power of the physician.

Medical sociology has been among the disciplines devoting themselves to encouraging patients to speak. Medical sociology has traditionally been preoccupied with defining patients' rights and patients' needs. As such it has been the most forthright of sociological specialties to describe itself as an "applied" discipline. It speaks against medical power in order to reform and improve medical practice. It teaches patients to speak against medical power in order to reform and improve medical practice. Recently medical sociology has divided itself into a sociology *of* medicine and a sociology *in* medicine.[1] Both subdisciplines place the highest value on the self that speaks about what is important to it. For the sociology of medicine, only the self that speaks about what is important to it can countermand the monopolistic tendency of medicine to define and control the rights of people as patients and citizens. For sociology in medicine the self must speak about what is important to it in order to convey information that may be crucial to the quality of medical care.[2]

Medical sociology's preoccupation with patients' rights and needs has, however, caused it to adopt a narrow perspective on the pervasive phenomenon of patients talking about themselves. It has tended to understand this phenomenon as a shift in the balance of power in the doctor-patient relationship. As the "classic" formulation of Szasz and Hollander would have it, there has been a shift from the "parent-infant" model of "activity-passivity" to the "adult-adult" model of "mutual participation."[3]

The way in which speaking about what is important is distributed between patient and physician may give insight into the "balance of power." But to examine this distribution is hardly to illuminate the phenomenon of patients seeking to speak about themselves. There is a more profound question to be asked than medical sociology has asked yet: In what terms are patients speaking about themselves? If you ask a class of medical sociology students how doctors ought to act toward patients, they will give you the same answers as a class of fourth-year medical students. They will speak more stridently than medical students, but their views on the proper conduct of the medical encounter will be the same as the views of doctors-to-be. Most "alternative health care" manuals do not differ significantly from medical textbooks in the terms in which they frame their arguments for proper care. The "debate" over the proper conduct of childbirth has been conducted in the terms of obstetrics for nearly 200 years even though obstetrics' terms for conducting the debate have changed over time. Might it be that patients and all who think they are rebelling against medicine are speaking in the same terms as medicine? And, if patients and physicians speak in the same terms about what is important, what does that say about changing relations of power in medicine?

For the most part, medical sociology has not approached the phenomenon of the self beginning to speak about itself by inquiring into the particular nature of the terms in which patients speak. That is, medical sociology has not been concerned with how patients think of themselves or how patients objectify themselves. The discipline has not been concerned with the rules of language that tell patients how to speak convincingly or truthfully about the self. It has not been concerned with the rules that make possible all those books that instruct us how to speak the truth. Since medical sociology has not concerned itself with these problems, it has not been able to ask truly probing questions about the significance that the process of the self creating itself as an object has for the self's relations of power with medicine.

The work of Michel Foucault has drawn our attention to questions that medical sociology has not addressed or cannot address. Foucault tells us that the goal of his work "has been to create a history of the different modes by which, in our culture, human beings are made subjects." His work has dealt with "modes of objectification which transform human beings into subjects."[4] One mode directly addresses medicine and its theoretical infrastructure: "the objectivizing of the sheer fact of being alive in natural history or biology."[5] What has recently come to be the focus of Foucault's studies is very much germane to the question of understanding how the terms in which patients speak about themselves are linked to changing structures of medical power, namely, his study of the "way a human being turns himself into a subject."[6]

It is thus Foucault's work and not medical sociology that provides the most productive starting point from which to grasp the meaning of the contemporary phenomenon of patients coming out of the shadows to speak about what is important to them. To undertake our task we do not have to engage in the seemingly interminable question of locating Foucault's work in the intellectual currents of our times. Nor do we have to use, or even understand, his "archeology of knowledge" method of which, as far as we can tell, he is the sole practitioner. To treat his work as a starting point is to see it as no more, but equally as no less, than being "of overriding interest."[7]

What is of overriding interest is the way Foucault has given new life to the old aphorism "knowledge is power." Medical sociology tends to treat medical knowledge as simply a technical knowledge about the facts of nature. Starting from an "empiricist model of medical knowledge and clinical practice" in which "meaning attaches to basic utterances in a language through a conventional association between a 'language element' and a given 'world element,' "[8] medical sociology shows little interest in the constitutive properties of medical language. This is strange since the idea that language objectifies things and constitutes a world about which it then becomes possible for us to speak as a "real world" is not an alien idea to sociology.[9] Sociology understands that there are rules that govern the distinction between the "real" and the "imaginary." These are not rules that we learn in schools or in books, but we "know" them nonetheless. They permit us to conduct a discourse that can stake a claim to "speaking true" about the world. Foucault's work commends itself to us as a starting point because it focuses attention on the rules for speaking true that govern the medical discourse.

The medical discourse is a discourse on life and death. It is more than just a set of facts known by physicians and embodied in a professional, specialized, inaccessible language. The medical discourse is a set of rules that enables facts to become facts for both physicians and patients. It is a set of rules that covers not only what is important to doctors but also what patients can speak about as important. Knowledge is power precisely because the knowledge embedded in the medical discourse supplies rules by which patients ascertain when they are speaking true about the self and when they are speaking about things that are imaginary. Knowledge tells the person what is important and not fanciful about his or her experience of illness and patienthood. Contrary to the view of medical sociology, the person does not dissolve the activity of power as he or she begins to speak about what is important. Invoking knowledge about what is important to the person *is* the activity of power:

> In a society such as ours, but basically in any society, there are manifold relations of power which permeate, characterize and constitute the social body, and these relations of power cannot themselves be established, consolidated nor implemented without the production, accumulation, circulation and functioning of a discourse. . . . We must speak the truth; we are constrained or condemned to confess or to discover the truth. Power never ceases its interrogation, its inquisition, its registration of the truth: it institutionalizes, professionalizes and rewards its pursuit. In the last analysis, we must produce truth as we must produce wealth, indeed, we must produce truth in order to produce wealth in the first place.

In another way, we are also subjected to truth in the sense
in which it is the truth that makes the laws, that produces
the true discourse which, at least partially, decides, trans-
mits and itself extends upon the effects of power. In the
end, we are judged, condemned, classified, determined
in our undertakings, destined to a certain mode of living
or dying, as a function of the true discourses which are
the bearers of the specific effects of power.[10]

If we begin to interpret the phenomenon of patients speaking
about things that are important to them, we run the risk of turning
treasured notions on their heads. Patients' speech may not penetrate the medical discourse; patients' speech may only penetrate
what patients say about themselves. We may have to suspend the
seemingly self-evident idea that to study power we must focus on
exclusionary practices. Instead of asking why medicine tries to
keep patients alienated in the medical encounter (as, self-evidently
it does, so the argument would go), we may have to ask why
medicine has started including patients as partners in medical work.
We might have to understand power differently. "We must cease
once and for all," Foucault has said, "to describe the effects of
power in negative terms: it 'excludes,' it 'represses,' it 'censors,'
it 'abstracts,' it 'masks,' it 'conceals.' In fact, power produces; it
produces reality; it produces domains of objects and rituals of truth.
The individual and the knowledge that may be gained of him belong
to this production."[11] We may have to question our reflex-like pro-
clivity to understand patients' speaking about themselves as a rebellion against an immoral power. We may have to treat this modern
phenomenon, instead, as a different form of the play of power.

Medicine has changed significantly in the last three decades or
so. We have to open ourselves to the possibility that we are seeing
a great medical sermon that, like Foucault's "great sexual sermon,"
"has had its subtle theologians and its popular voices. . . ." We
may be living through a change in the medical discourse that "has
swept through our societies over the last decades . . . chastised

the old order, denounced hypocracy, and praised the rights of the immediate and the real [and] made people dream of a New City.''[12]

We do not deny that when patients speak about what is important to the self, they are resisting old repressions even though they might speak in a language shared by medicine. But we must go beyond this appealing, self-congratulatory image and examine whether they might not be dreaming a variant of the old dreams that have always been dreamt about New Cities where nothing wild can exist to upset the order of things. It requires no great subtlety to see between the lines of announcements of ''medical breakthroughs'' a dream about a New City that is not in some shadow world beyond this one, but that is in this world where the vicissitudes of life itself would at last be tamed. This book is about the link between this dream and the new play of medical power whose sign is the patient turning his speech toward himself.

# Two

# The Disappearance of the Experiencing Person

**M**EDICINE TODAY looks like a pentimento. *Pentimento* is the term used to describe those old paintings in which one image has been painted over another, but the overlying image is so thin that the one under it still shows through. Ghostly figures of small children, dogs or trees seep through into portraits or landscapes because the images meant to obscure them cannot obliterate them completely.

In today's medicine different images of the doctor and patient are intertangled, the new not absolutely clear, the old still discernible but no longer dominant. This pentimento-like character of medicine is most vivid where patients are undergoing those processes that bracket life: giving birth and dying. There is the old image of the woman confined to her labor room. She waits silently to be taken to the delivery room where she will be strapped to a table, flat on her back with her legs in stirrups. To her the obstetrician looks like a mannequin whose actions seem to be human actions but whose intentions behind the acts are opaque to her. She cannot read the meaning of those acts because she has no language, no dictionary, with which to interpret them or make sense of them. We still live with this image of birth, but there is a new one being superimposed over it. This is the figure of a woman wandering through a permeable space as she waits to give birth. She goes from family room, through the halls of the maternity ward, to the cafeteria, to the birthing room, all at will. She may even give birth at home with friends and neighbors near. She does not wait for the play of forces and counterforces to begin in her body. Her obstetrical parts are not isolated on the delivery table as if they had no meaning other than as objects of medical practice. She is involved in an experience for which nothing can be regarded as extraneous. She will have a family-centered, not a uterus-centered birth.

At the other end of life is the image of the patient waiting to die, oftentimes wishing for death and waging a silent and discreet war with the network of tubes and shunts that support life's processes. This is the patient whose wait seems painfully interminable because it depends on things that have no life of their own. This patient disseminates information in a myriad of forms, and that information is checked, monitored and observed, but the patient is held incommunicado. This remains, to a degree, our image of dying, but there is a new image being superimposed over it. This is the dying person who does not die in a painfully dense solitude, but who is acknowledged to be alive by the kind of human attention accorded to the living. Sometimes this person does not die as a patient but as a member of a family that assembles to witness his death. This person dies within a network of emotions and feelings that flow between the dying person and others in ways that would be indiscreet, embarrassing and disruptive were he a patient.

These pentimento-like images are such an integral part of the social discourse about contemporay medicine that it seems strange to ask about the character of the changes they represent. Their meaning seems self-evident. Aren't patients and potential patients liberating themselves from a technologically advanced form of medical care that has become indifferent to and even oppressive of the full scope of their humanness? Aren't the new images signs of successful struggle against medical domination? The language used by students of medical change tends to reflect the interpretation of medical history as a history of increasingly depersonalized care that is coupled with a politicized image of assertive, if not rebellious, patients. This language informs the commonplace discourses on today's medicine.

For example, the foreword to a new medical textbook called *The Patient: Biological Psychological, and Social Dimensions of Medical Practice* says: "The old-fashioned doctor, whose departure from the modern medical scene is so greatly lamented, was amply aware of each patient's personality, family, work, and way of life. Today, we often blame a doctor's absence of awareness on moral and ethical deficiency either in medical education or in the character of people who become physicians." The text continues, "An alternative explanation, however, is that doctors are just as moral, ethical, and concerned as ever before, but that a vast amount of additional new information has won the competition for attention. The data available to the old-fashioned doctor were a patient's history, physical examination and 'personal profile' together with a limited number of generally ineffectual therapeutic agents. A doctor today deals with an enormous array of additional new information, which comes from X rays, biopsies, cytology, electrographic tracings and the phantasmagoria of contemporary laboratory tests; and the doctor must also be aware of a list of therapeutic possibilities that are both more effective and far more extensive than ever before."[1] According to this history, the physician and the patient remain constant over time. The doctor remains moral and committed. The patient remains sick and seeking relief. Knowledge progresses and is manifest in the deployment of tests, diagnostic procedures and new, more effective therapies. A distinction is made, as another text put it, "between the 'science' and 'art' of medicine, with medicine centering itself" almost wholly on science.[2] The progress of medicine divides the patient among many specialties. The plethora of hard facts derived from medical inquiry gains the physician's attention and displaces from view all the personal aspects of a patient that were central to the medical encounter in the past. The doctor-patient relationship becomes more and more alienated but through no one's fault or conscious design.

Out of alienation, assertive patients have been able to fashion their liberation from an oppression almost like that of politics, this history tells us. In the old regime, as Bernard Barber points out, "the doctor is superordinate, the authority, sometimes a person to be venerated. The patient and others are subordinate, respectful, even deferential. The doctor is active, knowledgeable and secure in the system; the patient and others are passive, ill-informed, frightened and dependent." In the newly emerging order, "patients are not so much subordinates of the authoritative doctor, but more clearly partners, even 'quasi-colleagues.' . . . All participants are obligated to be knowledgeable, independent and active. Mutuality and reduction of inequality are preferred to one-sidedness and inequality."[3]

We believe that characterizing the changes medicine is undergoing in these terms is far too limiting and superficial. It is certainly true that today's technologically-oriented specialist wrestles with more information than yesterday's still venerated "old-fashioned doctor," but medicine itself does not mark the origin of its modernity with an increasing quantity of technological information that makes scientific theories about life and death possible. "Modern medicine," Foucault says, "has fixed its own date of birth in the first years of the eighteenth century. Reflecting on its situation, it identifies the origin of its positivity with a return—over and above all theory—to the modest but effecting level of the perceived."[4] What medicine reckons as the origin of its modernity was not an increase in the quantity of information available to it but a radical shift in the manner of simplifying information, a shift captured by Foucault's notion of a "return to the perceived." The development of a "gaze," an informed, purposeful look at life, set in motion the history of medicine that contemporary students wish to cast in terms of inexorable technological advances and confrontations between doctors and patients.

Reiser tells us that the physician at the beginning of the seventeenth century, prior to the development of the gaze, relied chiefly on three techniques to diagnose illness: "the patient's statement in words which described his symptoms; the physician's observations of signs of the illness, his patient's physical appearance and behavior; and more rarely, the physician's manual examination of the patient's body. Seventeenth and eighteenth century physicians generally used the word 'symptom' to mean any datum of clinical evidence that indicated any departure from good health. The term 'sign' generally denoted a symptom that provided special information to the physician: for instance, to indicate that a certain phenomenon of illness had occurred, or even might occur."[5] On the basis of the distinction between "symptom" and "sign," information about the patient's disease was dispersed across the full range of possibilities open to the pre-modern physician's experience of the patient. This included speaking with the patient. The physician involved himself in all the complexities of culling information from the flow of speech such as deciphering codes, filling in narrative gaps and making empathic leaps.

By the twentieth century the distinction between "symptom" and "sign" had vanished. "James MacKenzie in his 1920 book, *Symptoms and Their Interpretation,* used the words symptoms and signs interchangeably to mean 'a reaction of the tissues of the body to a noxious agent.' "[6] The rule for identifying the information needed to produce a truthful account of disease had become simplified even though the information needed had become a complex mass in its own right. Signs and symptoms both originated in tissues. The rule physicians had to follow to gain information was "look into the body and see the disease." Beyond this rule there was nothing that could be called necessary information. The patient's speech about his experience of his body and the physician's experience of the patient disappeared from the medical encounter. Medicine developed a studied indifference to the person experiencing illness.

The rule "look and see" follows from Morgagni's notion that anatomical lesions "not only provoke the maladies, but are also responsible for their intrinsic differences."[7] "Look and see" was the rule Bichat (1801) knew would make medicine "modern": "You may take notes for twenty years, from morning to night at the bedside of the sick . . . and all will be to you only a confusion of symptoms, which, not being united in one point, will necessarily present only a train of incoherent phenomena. Open up a few bodies; this obscurity will soon disappear, which observation alone would never have been able to dissipate."[8]

For today's physician, Morgagni's and Bichat's notion of there being a single point in the body which, when seen by the physician, unifies disparate signs and symptoms into the truth of disease, is naive. But the rule that directs the gaze into the body (for that is where information lies that allows the physician to speak the truth) has remained constant over the 200 years since Morgagni and Bichat announced it in their medical treatises. This rule structures the modern medical discourse by establishing the identities of the patient, the doctor and the disease.

Because the patient only lives his or her body and cannot see the information it yields about the truth of disease, the patient's suffering can only be confused suffering no matter how articulate he or she may be in speaking about symptoms and sensations. Thus a patient, Alice Stewart Trillin, stricken with cancer, writes in 1981 in *The New England Journal of Medicine:* "Whenever I am threatened by panic my doctor sits me down and tells me something concrete. He draws a picture of my lungs, or my lymph nodes; he explains as well as he can how cancer cells work and what might be happening in my body. Together we approach my disease intelligently and rationally, as a problem to be solved, an exercise in logic to be worked out. . . . Through knowledge, through medicine, through intelligence we do have some control."[9]

It is somewhat fanciful but not untrue to think of Morgagni and Bichat as urging on medicine the logo it eventually adopted as a sign of its modernity: the picture of the anatomy lesson. Indeed, the notion that the anatomy lesson serves as modern medicine's logo is not at all fanciful when we consider how often we see reproductions of the frontispiece of Vesalius's *De Humani Corporis Fabrica* (Plates 2.1 and 2.2) on the walls of places where medicine does its work. Choulant, in 1852, described the frontispiece of *De*

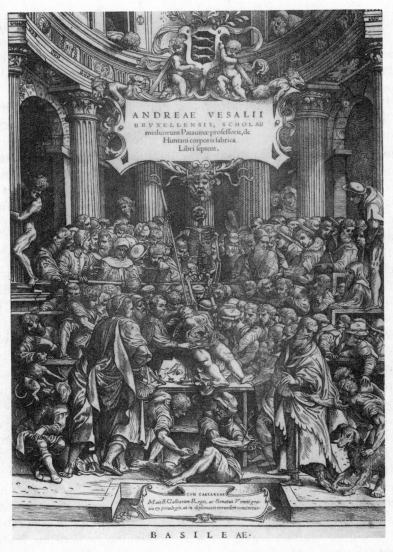

PLATE 2.1  Frontispiece from Vesalius, *De Fabrica*, 1545 edition. Courtesy of Dana Biomedical Library, Dartmouth Medical School.

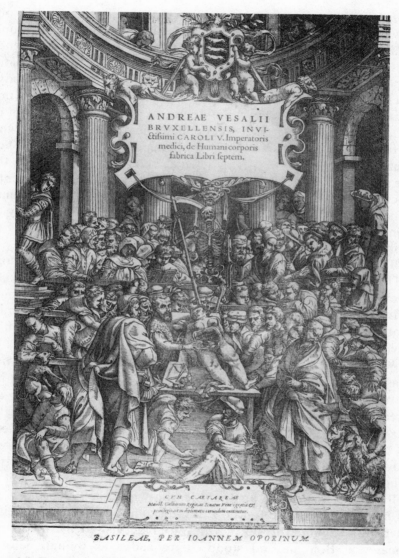

**PLATE 2.2** Frontispiece from Vesalius, *De Fabrica,* 1653 edition.

*Fabrica* with an anatomical precision that Vesalius no doubt would have applauded: "Vesalius standing beside a dissecting table upon which there lies a female body with the abdominal cavity opened; Vesalius's left hand with the forefinger raised, his right hand holding a pointer and resting upon the cadaver; at the head of the body a skeleton standing erect with a long staff in its right hand. Surrounding these is a large assembly of people of different classes. On the left, in the window, stands a nude man clinging to a column, while at the bottom on the right, we see a living dog brought in."[10] Choulant's purified and objectifying language conveys, to a degree, that we are looking at a public display of medical virtuosity. Apparently, such public dissections were not uncommon during the Renaissance.[11] What Choulant's language does not convey is the way the configuration of this great piece of Renaissance art identifies the principal elements of modern medicine.

That particular anatomy lesson is well chosen as medicine's logo. "The *Fabrica*," Reiser says, "was not a book that merely corrected previous anatomical errors. More important, it announced a new principle of fact-finding and truth-testing in anatomy: all anatomical statements and hypotheses were to be subjected to a methodical review by the dissections and observation of human cadavers. . . ."[12]

Whether Vesalius knew it or not, the frontispiece of the *Fabrica* was to become the lodestone that would lead medicine to its modernity. It articulated an ideology that grounds the visions and dreams of medicine. It was, as Vesalius wrote in presenting the book to the Emperor Charles V, "an account from which we learn of the body and of the mind and furthermore of a certain divine power consisting of the harmony of both, in sum of ourselves, whom to know is man's proper study."[13] Harvey Cushing felt the full significance of the anatomy lesson when, in 1900, barely out of medical school, he toured Europe as any well-educated gentleman was expected to do. On that tour he visited the anatomical theater at Bologna and stood "bareheaded as though before a shrine."[14] Modern medicine has adopted the anatomy lesson as its logo and elevated its image to such a level that even without the cast of characters present, Harvey Cushing would feel compelled to venerate one place where such demonstrations were conducted.

Cushing was not venerating a new technology. Teaching anatomy from human cadavers had been going on since the beginning of the fourteenth century.[15] He was venerating something else that modern medicine identified as the mark of its modernity. This "mark" is the rule for knowing the truth of disease that has nourished modern medicine for 200 years. As Georges Canguilhem put it, "disease plays its tricks at the tissue level and in this sense, there can be sickness without a sick person."[16] The frontispiece to Vesalius's *Fabrica* is not the first depiction of an anatomy lesson, but its particular configuration rests on the principle stated by the French physician René Leriche in 1936: "If one wants to define disease it must be dehumanized. . . . In disease, when all is said and done, the least important thing is man."[17] In effect, the power of the medical discourse and the modern medical discourse as power were born when the experiencing person was displaced by the rule "look and see." This rule simultaneously defined what it was possible to say that was true about disease and prevented the person living with disease from saying anything about it.

"Looking" dominates the frontispiece of the *Fabrica*. There is first of all what is being looked at: death in the form of the silent, anonymous cadaver. The cadaver is the central figure of this picture. Its abdomen has been opened so that everyone can peer in and see; it is as if death itself had been put on display. Lest there be any mistake that it is death that is to be seen, a faceless skeleton points toward the open abdomen. Second, there is Vesalius. He is an instantly distinguishable figure. He does not look like the crowd, nor does he look into the cadaver. He looks out at us as if he were extending an invitation. We cannot mistake Vesalius for any one of the figures that press in on the dissecting table, for he is the one person in the scene who knows already what is to be seen. Although Vesalius literally stands out in the crowd, the artist has not made too much of him, and neither must we. There is not a single figure in the picture looking at Vesalius. Except for a few who are otherwise distracted, everyone is looking directly past Vesalius into the open abdominal cavity where he points. Vesalius, while important, is not central. The anatomy lesson is a spectacle without a performer, a spectacle with a dead star. Vesalius is interchangeable with anyone else who, knowing what is to be seen, stands and instructs those who wish to see.[18]

Medicine reads itself in this woodcut. It is busy and complicated in form but also deceptively simple in theme: the picture elevates the dead body from the "lowest of the low," to use Cassirer's phrase,[19] and says that if it is the truth of man that we seek to know, then that truth will be disclosed only when we make everything about him visible.

Medicine does not hang the anatomy lesson on its walls simply because it depicts a technology for collecting knowledge. More significant, it was a harbinger of the revolutionary dictum that informs medical work: nothing has the right to resist the need to see and to know. It would be a mistake to lose sight of the fact that the frontispiece consists of men looking into the body of a woman. On the basis of its new dictum, medicine moved into areas of life from which it had been barred previously. Medicine made childbirth a part of its domain.[20] Medicine could do anything, including violation of all social rules of modesty and decorum, if it could be made to seem in the medical interests of the patient to do so.[21] Vesalius opened the corpse in an act of violent intrusion into the intimate and private. But modern medicine adopts this picture as its logo because it depicts the apocryphal moment from which point forward all of its acts are privileged from ever being characterized as violent intrusions again. If medicine is called to do something, there is nothing that can limit its knowing. Its doing must follow Leonardo's dictum: "To lie is so vile that even if it were in speaking well of Godly things, it would take off something of God's grace, and Truth is so excellent that if it praises but small things, they become noble. . . . But you who live in dreams are better pleased with sophistical reasons and frauds of wit in great and uncertain things than with those reasons which are certain and natural and not so far above us.''[22]

The anatomy lesson brings the corpse into close conjunction with the living body, from which it was once radically separated. Life and death are joined together under a single discourse, but in a special way that merits attention. The nude figure clinging to the column in the upper left of the woodcut is probably the live model on which Vesalius illustrated external anatomy during the same lesson he displayed the internal anatomy of the corpse. The figure looks like he would flee the scene if possible, but he cannot. The anatomy lesson locked his vitality in the same scene with death. Yet this figure is the only one in the entire picture that is artistically barred from its central area. The lighting of the scene creates a gulf of white between the nude and the rest of the action. Compelled to be part of the scene even though terrified and yet barred from participating in it fully, this person who represents medicine's patient has been trapped in this untenable position by the force of medical logic for over 400 years.

It took more than 200 years for the connection between the living and the dead to bear the fruit which we now identify as modern medicine. Early clinical anatomy identified disease and death with alterations in the shape and surfaces of organs, but not until 1761 did anyone take the crucial step of suggesting that hidden anatomic changes could be detected in the living patient. Leopold Auenbrugger anticipated this fundamental principle of diagnosis in his pamphlet *Inventum Novum* in 1761. His idea lay dormant for another 50 years until it was rediscovered by Covisart and set in its place as a cornerstone of modern medicine.[23] Medicine built quickly and steadily on the link between structural alterations observed in the anatomy theater and symptoms observed at the bedside. Every advance—the microscope, the X ray, and so on—probed the body more deeply and revealed finer and finer structures.

We need to understand the history of modern medicine as a history of restructurings of a discourse on life and death. After the appearance of modern medicine late in the eighteenth century the relationship between life and death would no longer be represented by the imaginary figures of a *danse macabre* where "in the shape of his body Everyman carries his own death with him and dances with it through his life."[24] The relationship between life and death would now be depicted in figures that represent what Reiser calls the "body's vivifying activities,"[25] figures that are no longer efficacious metaphors but an array of numbers, charts, graphs and words in the medical record that record the reality that discloses itself to the medical gaze. Everything that is possible to say about the truth of both life and death is exhausted in a discourse on the visible. Anything else that could be said is relegated to the domain of the imaginative where language evokes images that are as thin as smoke.

The first restructuring of the discourse on life and death is present in the two premises established by the great eighteenth century anatomist, Morgagni. Reiser states them thus: "First, disease often leaves telltale footprints on the tissues of the body; second, study of these footprints is the best way for physicians to verify judgments made on the living, and the key to achieving clinical excellence. . . . Morgagni's appeal to the physician [was] to examine the structural changes wrought by disease on the body's inner fabric. . . ."[26] From the anatomist's viewpoint the "telltale footprints" left by diseases are the means for tracking the visible history of death in the body, and the diseases that leave these visible tracks define death's polymorphous face.

Modern medicine created an empirics of death. Death could be observed precisely at the point where the observable history of a disease ends the life that harbored it. "Death is therefore multiple and dispersed in time: it is not that absolute privileged point at which time stops and moves back; like disease itself, it has a teeming presence that analysts may divide into time and space. . . ."[27]

The medical gaze maps and charts this teeming presence as the multiple but specific paths followed by death in the body. Thus "life, disease and death now form a technical and conceptual trinity." The medical gaze is like "the gaze of an eye that has seen death—a great white eye that unties the knot of life."[28]

This conceptual trinity has a structure, a horizon on which everything related to it becomes ordered. "Life" gains a specificity that shuns metaphysics. The medical discourse on life became a discourse on the mechanisms that account for the "vital capacities" of the body.[29] To know life is to specify the basal force and energies essential to understanding the structures and functions of the body. The scientific challenge is to know the identity of life in terms of what is "normal" to it. The word "normal" first appeared in 1759 and the word "normalized" in 1834.[30] "In the course of the nineteenth century," Canguilhem says, "the real identity of normal and pathological vital phenomena, apparently so different, and given opposing values by human experience, became a kind of scientifically guaranteed dogma. . . ."[31] It was, Foucault points out, "the chemical operation, which, by isolating the component elements, made it possible to define the composition, to establish common points, resemblances and differences with other totalities, and thus to found a classification that was no longer based on specific types but on forms of relations."[32] Life became a produced life—a problem to be dissected, differentiated, identified and classified in terms of the lawful characteristics of the energies that produced the normal.

Because death was a visible history of disease that could be reconstructed in its entirety by starting with the body whose life disease ended, death became the opposition to life. Death became the negative space that gave life its shape. "Life," said Bichat, "is the sum of all the functions by which death is resisted."[33]

The modern discourse about disease did not arise as a discourse about an abstract value assigned to a visible deviation from the "normal." Disease, Foucault suggests, was "the active subject that exercises [analysis, division, separation, and so on] pitilessly upon the organism. If the disease is to be analyzed, it is because it is itself analysis; an ideological decomposition can only be the repetition in the doctor's consciousness of the decomposition raging in the patient's body."[34] Modern medical language admits disease to reality as a force that rends, shreds apart and decomposes the integrity of life. From the moment of its origin until now, modern medicine looks at death, seeing in it those "forms and deformations, figures and accidents . . . displaced, destroyed or modified elements bound together in sequence according to a geography that can be followed step by step. . . ."[35]

By the end of the eighteenth century, disease could no longer be understood as a disturbance of a "harmony" and "equilibrium" that was nature.[36] At that point in history, disease changes from "disequilibrium and discordance" or "an effort on the part of nature to effect a new equilibrium in man"[37] into "a polemical situation: either a battle between the organism and a foreign substance, or an internal struggle between opposing forces."[38]

Birth itself, the beginning of a life, fell under that polemic and was admitted to the practice of medical discourse as a strange sort of pathology. Birth, like death, was once a momentous event because, as a threshold across which life entered, it was also a moral event. "Birth was a moral crisis through which women had to pass. That is to say, the delivering woman's behavior in birth was thought to reveal her moral character."[39] The barber-surgeon, an embryonic form of the modern surgeon, was ancillary to the event of birth. He was called upon to use his "hooks, knives, levers, saws and other tools to pull a fetus from the womb either whole or in parts" when midwives deemed it necessary.[40] The midwife attended an event whose momentous nature lay in being revelatory. "If the child had not been fathered by a woman's husband, it was thought that during her labor pains or during expulsion she might shout out the name of the real father. A child born dead or anomalous might be taken as a reflection of the mother's and perhaps even the father's low moral standing or diminished stature in the sight of God. But even the moral crisis of childbirth was 'natural.' The moral crisis of birth was simply one manifestation of humankind's standing in relationship to God and of woman's inferior standing in society. It was, in other words, one aspect of the natural order and one aspect of the nature of women.''[41]

By the mid-eighteenth century, ''systematic observation of birth which the hospital allowed proceeded apace and culminated in . . . pelvimetry—instrumental measurement of the female pelvis.''[42] Life had become identified with specific structures and functions of the body and the pathological was identified with deviations from normative states, displays of the various ways the body decomposes through the action of disease. The machine became the compelling metaphor for the body. ''Each part of the body was a machine unto itself and a component of a larger machine.''[43] The profession of obstetrics originates with and forms itself around the tool that addresses the machine. The physician, before he is anything else, stands as the chief spectator before a polemic in nature no longer constituted as a moral polemic but as a play of force and counterforce, movement and resistance. In the first two decades of the twentieth century, two leading obstetricians, Ralph Pomeroy and Joseph B. DeLee, sum it all up with regard to birth. Pomeroy called the fetal head a ''battering ram'' which ''shatter[s] a resisting outlet,'' and arguing for the use of episiotomies, he asked rhetorically, ''why not open the gates and close them after the procession has passed?''[44] DeLee employs the mechanical metaphor for other purposes. He ''believed that a woman should be as 'anatomically perfect' after delivery as she was before and that since birth was a process where the fetal 'head has been pounding and grinding the muscle like a piece of steak is pounded by a mallet' an episiotomy was the only way to preserve the vaginal entrance and restore 'virginal conditions.' ''[45] DeLee, paraphrasing Bichat, knew that life's standards were revealed by the malignant forces that seek to twist and deform it.

The language of modern medicine bears two parallel themes. First, it understands life as the constellation of essential forces and substances that produce it, and second, it understands itself as a force that counters those energies and substances that produce a visible history of violence in the body and that end life. These themes remain constant through time but they have been recast in somewhat different terms. Today it is less a matter of seeing life as virginally pure, invaded by blindly hostile diseases, than it is of seeing disease as something coiled at the very heart of life. Foucault points out the concept of "error" has become biomedically crucial. "For at life's most basic level, the play of code and decoding leaves room for chance, which, before being disease, deficit or monstrosity, is something like a perturbation in the information system, something like a 'mistake.' In the extreme, life is what is capable of error."[46] This is exactly the concept used by a medical scientist at a seminar on gout: "Here nature made a mistake . . . similar to the mistake she made with the vermiform appendix. There is no good reason for the body to produce so much uric acid."[47] If the nature of the truth spoken by medicine has changed somewhat, the structure of that truth has remained constant. Both life and its opposite—disease and death—are the activities of mindless forces of nature. The role of the physician is to make a mindless nature mindful of what reason sees, reflects, and speaks as true about life.

Modern medicine organizes itself around a specific kind of awe of the body, an awe conveyed in its logo. The philosopher Jacob Needleman tells of his experience as a premedical student assisting in a hospital autopsy room: "I was cutting two, sometimes four corpses a day. At the same time, I was reading every medical book I could get hold of. From everything I understood in these medical texts, and from what I saw everyday with my own eyes and heard from the doctors who patiently answered all my questions, I found myself facing an intolerable contradiction. The human body, my human body, was so marvelously constructed, so complexly unified, so resilient, so intelligently adapted in the interrelationship of its parts with respect to the world around it, that it was incredible it should ever die at all. But for the same reasons it was equally incredible that it should continue to live more than a fraction of a second in a universe whose basic make-up was so alien to it."[48]

This "contradiction" is the same one reflected in obstetrical language from the moment obstetrics brought the awesome event of birth under its aegis as a marvelous process simultaneously fraught with impossibility.

No other kind of practice could be organized around such an awe of the body made visible, around this "intolerable contradiction," than a practice directed toward a governance of nature. "To govern disease," Canguilhem observes, "means to become acquainted with its relations with the normal state, which the living man—loving life—wants to regain. Hence the theoretical need, but a past due technique, to establish a scientific pathology by linking it to physiology."[49] But even before such a scientific pathology existed, indeed, as the very possibility for its existence, was Sydenham's thought in the mid-seventeenth century "that in order to help a sick man, his sickness had to be delimited and determined."[50] To acquire the power to govern nature, the medical gaze had, first, to become a gaze with the power to isolate, localize, circumscribe, and delimit.

The notion of "governing nature" is really too general and too mild to capture what passed between medicine and nature for almost two hundred years and continues to do so in many ways today. Mindless force is made mindful by opposing force with force. Knowledge becomes a force made manifest in the hands and instruments of the physician. The medical gaze, which at first blush is something passive that falls on a passive object, becomes a force that opposes force. It dedicates itself, Foucault notes, "to the endless task of absorbing experience in its entirety, and of mastering it."[51]

This language is a warlike language. It is true, as Susan Sontag has observed, that "the military metaphor in medicine first came into wide use in the 1880s, with the identification of bacteria as agents of disease. Bacteria were said to 'invade' or 'infiltrate.' " It is also true that the "talk of siege and war to describe disease now has, with cancer, a striking literalness and authority. Not only is the clinical course of the disease and its medical treatment thus described, but the disease itself is conceived as the enemy on which society wages war."[52] But this language of war came into existence at the original moment when medicine said that the face of death was constituted by the swollen, discolored and corrupted organs in the body that made visible the decomposition of the structures and functions of life. Foucault describes the moment this way: "Behind the doctor's back, death remained the great dark threat in which his knowledge and skill were abolished; it was the risk not only of life and disease but of knowledge that questioned them. With Bichat, the medical gaze pivots on itself and demands of death an account of life and disease, of its definitive immobility of their time and movements."[53]

In adopting the anatomy lesson as its logo, modern medicine identified itself with a discourse about life and death whose power lay not in conducting a dialogue with another, but in the capacity to speak to another who must listen silently if he wants to hear the truth spoken. In the anatomy lesson Vesalius conducts a spectacle and not a seminar. The spectacle is one-sided and devoid of a need for dialogue. The frontispiece of the *Fabrica* is medicine's cachet for the beginning of the end of the physician as discussant.

In the anatomy lesson there may be points to be clarified, facts to be sorted out, but there is no ambiguity to be discussed. The cadaver lies open before everyone. Regardless of one's point of view, one is compelled to see the same thing as everyone else in the room. When Vesalius points into the body, he reconciles every diverse perspective throughout the theater—a theater filled with "people of different classes" we are told—into a common focus called Truth. One must be taught to see it of course. That is why Vesalius instructs. When Vesalius speaks, he speaks to indicate. His words become inseparable from the things they signify.

Modern medicine employs a logo that situates the patient in a field of power characterized "by the minute but decisive change," to use Foucault's terms, "whereby the question: 'What is the matter with you?' . . . was replaced by that other question: 'Where does it hurt?' in which we recognize the operation of the clinic and the principle of its entire discourse."[54] The physician's task is to extract from the hidden recesses of the body signs of the disease that lies within. Symptoms are effect-signs pointing to their causes waiting to be seen. Once these signs are in hand, the physician can look for and then speak about the true nature of what causes them. Modern medicine sees its origin in the forging of "a new alliance . . . between words and things, enabling one *to see* and *to say*."[55] This is an alliance that subtracts the patient as an experiencing person from his body, the object that carries all the relevant information that yields the truth of his confused suffering.

The language of the patient interferes with those words which "with [their] qualitative precision, direct our gaze into a world of constant visibility."[56] Physicians would no longer need to engage their patient in dialogue. All that is important, indeed all that is real, would lie before the physician to be seen. Like Chekhov's physician, Doctor Andrew Ephimich Raghin, who found in the psychopathic ward an ill but "interesting young man" with whom he talked only to have his friends commit him to the same ward for conversing with a lunatic, physicians who try to engage their patients in discussions open themselves to suspicion and censure from their colleagues.[57] The whole of modern clinical experience was made possible by the rule of "look and see" the truth. "One could at last hold a scientifically structured discourse about an individual,"[58] an individual who might as well be dead given the extent of his or her participation in that discourse.

We should not think of the changes in medicine that we are living through today as a rebellion against the runaway growth of medical technology. These changes are the insertion of the experiencing person back into medical discourse. The person starting to reappear in medicine is not quite the same person who was excluded by the rule that equipped medicine to speak the truth of a person's suffering, but it is a person we will recognize just the same.

The history of dying reveals how the experiencing person suffered the most profound loss of himself to medicine around the turn of the eighteenth century. And in the recent history of dying we shall see how that loss, however much it appears on the surface that it is being reclaimed by the dying person as if he were storming the Bastille, is in reality being given back to him by the medical discourse itself. Dying is like a lightning rod that captures all the tensions into today's pentimento-like medicine.

## Three

## The Return of the Experiencing Person

THROUGH HIS SPEECH to sick patients the modern physician performed what Michael Balint insightfully called the "apostolic function": "It was almost as if every doctor had revealed knowledge of what was right and what was wrong for patients to expect and to endure, and further as if he had a sacred duty to convert to his faith all the ignorant and unbelieving among his patients."[1] For the dying, however, there was no revealing of knowledge, no evangelizing or performing of conversions. There was only the refusal to speak about death. Ironically, when medicine seized the right to speak the truth about death, no one spoke about it at all. When medicine made death visible, we could only think in terms of visible diseases conducting war against life. Death itself was never spoken about. A patient could say nothing about his dying because all his experience could represent was a confused subjectivity over the horror and ugliness that accompanied the end stage of a disease. The visible history of disease that ended life, about which physicians spoke, exhausted everything that could be said about the truth of dying. Medicine thought it a kindness to alleviate the patient's confusion by never speaking about dying.

Only recently, about 1970 by one reckoning, did physicians in the United States begin to tell their patients they were suffering from an illness that would almost certainly kill them.[2] It is in the history of the manner of our dying that we can see most vividly how modern physicians identified themselves with the kind of truth-speaking depicted in the anatomy lesson. And it is in the current manner of our dying that we begin to appreciate the fact that the patient's subjective experience, confused though it might have been since the end of the eighteenth century, is being reinserted into the medical encounter.

Philippe Ariès, in his monumental history of dying in the Western world, sees Tolstoi's Ivan Ilyich as a convenient symbol for how we came to die once it became unthinkable to die except as a patient. Ivan Ilyich places responsibility for the truth of his condition in the hands of his doctor. "His illness is suddenly a case that has a separate existence and must have a name. What name? It is up to the doctor to say it, and then he will know whether or not it is serious. For there are categories of illness that are dangerous and others that are benign. Everything depends on the diagnosis."[3] Ilyich's confused experience can only be resolved by a disease's name that only the doctor knows. Everything is ambiguous, and as Ilyich gets worse he keeps his warning pain to himself and from himself. "He does not give way; he guards his secret suffering, for fear of worrying those around him and also of giving the thing he feels swelling inside him greater reality by naming it."[4] Everybody including Ilyich colludes in a conspiracy never to speak the name and what it denotes: death. But the conspiracy is blown when Ilyich "overhears a conversation between his wife and his brother-in-law. 'But don't you see that he is dead?' the brother-in-law exclaims brutally. This is something new. Ilyich did not know, nor did his wife probably that this is how people see him."[5] His doctor clearly saw him this way, but he was the cardinal figure in the conspiracy. But even he cannot help communicating a sign which Ilyich is able to read about his dying. "Ivan Ilyich suddenly understands that he is going to die. 'The kidney, the appendix,' he thinks. 'No, that's not the point, it's a matter of life . . . or death. It is death, and here I am thinking about the appendix!' "[6] Ilyich thinks about dying and his doctor thinks about the disease and neither speaks about death. Everything deteriorates into bad farce.

"The doctor lends himself to the farce. He seems to be saying, 'You are upsetting yourself over nothing. We'll fix you up in no time.' Even after the final consultation with important specialists, and in spite of the aggravation of his condition, 'everyone was afraid to suddenly dissipate the correct lie and to let in so much reality.' "[7]

Why mask the unnameable reality in a dissimulating rhetoric and impose a taboo of silence on the word "death"? Because the word admits a welter of useless emotions—denial, fear, anger. It painfully upsets everybody, including the doctor, and makes the doctor's work more difficult. To avoid this messy situation became even more urgent fifty years or so after Tolstoi's story, as almost everyone came to the hospital to die. The subjective experience of dying became a potential disruption to routines and procedures needed in the medical workplace.[8] The medical workplace was devoted to prolonging life by keeping the history of disease from ending it. Death could not be admitted, even in name.

Ivan Illich and Philippe Ariès have both traced the history of this subtraction of the experiencing person from his dying. This descent into a taboo of silence is the allegory of the birth of modern medicine.

Philippe Ariès constructs the early history of western attitudes toward death as a movement from "tamed death" to death that "has become wild." He writes, "I do not mean that death had once been wild and that it has ceased to be so. I mean, on the contrary, that today it has become wild."[9] Ivan Illich, in his different but parallel history of attitudes toward death, suggests a similar direction of change when he observes: "We have seen death turn from God's call into a 'natural' event and later into a 'Force of nature.' . . . Death had paled into a metaphorical figure, and killer diseases had taken its place."[10] The history of death, as outlined by Ariès and Illich, exists in two phases which together point to a paradox: Once dying was everywhere visible and death was invisible but tamed; later, dying became invisible and death everywhere visible but wild.

For millennia the dying person had a visible and public identity. Dying was a public event. In fact, "right up to the end, everything took place according to a schedule that was arranged by the dying person himself."[11] For thousands of years it was the secret or sudden death that was unspeakable: "a sudden death was a vile and ugly death; it was frightening; it seemed a strange and monstrous thing that nobody dared talk about."[12]

Until the thirteenth century, death and life were intermingled. They did not stand in opposition to each other. "The spectacle of the dead, whose bones were always being washed up to the surface of the cemeteries, as was the skull in Hamlet, made no more impression upon the living than did the idea of their own death. They were as familiar with the dead as they were familiarized with the idea of their own death."[13] This "familiarity with death is a form of acceptance of the order of nature, an acceptance which can be both naive, in day-to-day affairs, and learned in astrological speculations. In death man encountered one of the great laws of the species, and he had no thought of escaping it or glorifying it. He merely accepted it with just the proper amount of solemnity due one of the important thresholds which each generation always had to cross."[14] The crossing of that threshold was marked by solemn ceremonies and rituals that conveyed the inextricable intertwining of death with life, of the invisible with the visible. Illich writes: "From the fourth century onwards, the church struggled against a pagan tradition in which crowds, naked, frenzied and brandishing swords, danced on the tombs in the churchyard. . . . For a thousand years Christian churches and cemeteries remained dance floors. Death was an occasion for the renewal of life."[15]

In the late middle ages death takes on a different order of familiarity—a macabre intimacy that arises with a self-consciousness that death stands outside life, separate from it, and not constitutive of its very texture and fabric. The reality of death becomes the reality "of one's own death" to use Ariès's phrase.[16] "During the second half of the Middle Ages, from the twelfth to the fifteenth centuries, three categories of mental images were brought together: the image of death, that of the individual's knowledge of his own biography, and that of the passionate attachment for things and creatures possessed during one's lifetime. Death became the occasion when man was most able to reach an awareness of himself."[17]

Dancing on the dead disappears and is replaced by figures dancing with death. Death, Illich points out, "was transformed into a meditative, introspective experience."[18] By the end of the fifteenth-century, "death has become an independent figure who calls each man, woman, and child, first as a messenger from God but soon insisting on his own sovereign rights."[19] Each human can identify himself in Holbein's *Danse Macabre* in the embrace of a faceless death that comes to him from a point outside the world "as the egalitarian executioner of a law that whirls everyone along and then mows them down. From a lifelong encounter, death has turned into the event of a moment."[20]

After the twelfth century, great ceremonies and rituals arose to tame a death that was an "event of a moment." Death, then self-consciously encountered as a personal fate, was no longer part of the natural order but was, instead, a thing subject to ordering. Ceremonies and rituals ordered matters and thereby prepared one to die. The attitude of "familiar simplicity toward death" took on a ceremonial form "which [was] to last until the end of the nineteenth century. The dying person must be the center of a group of people."[21]

People did not simply gather to witness a dying; they staged a ceremonial dying. The dying man spoke of a premonition he had received of his impending death. Ariès is at pains to point out that the premonition, as miraculous as it might seem to us, "was an absolutely natural phenomenon, even when it was accompanied by wonders."[22] By making known to others "the fact that death made itself known in advance,"[23] the dying man invoked the ceremonial practices that conferred on him a new identity. We see such ceremonies already formed in oral epics such as the *Chanson de Roland*. "The acts performed by the dying man, once he has been warned that his end is near, have a ceremonial ritual quality. We recognize these acts as the still-oral source for what later became the medieval testament, which was required by the church as part of the last sacrament: the profession of faith, the confession of sins, the pardon of survivors, the pious dispositions on their behalf, the commendation of one's soul to God, the choice of burial."[24]

The ceremonial staging of dying expressed a complex of concepts that constituted a social discourse in whose terms death and the dying person were known. This discourse was not conducted by a single social class in a single historical period, but pervades Western history from at least "the knight in the *Chanson*" to "those peasants in the heart of Russia whom Solzhenitsyn describes in *The Cancer Ward*."[25] Clearly the dominant form of the discourse was Christian, but Ariès wants us to see beyond that: "Christianity adopted the traditional ideas of ordinary people and Stoic philosophers about the gradual deterioration of the human body from the moment of birth."[26] Christianity arose as an expression of one of the "ideas about continuation [that] form a foundation that is common to all the ancient religions and to Christianity."[27] Christianity, with its "idea of an immortal soul, the seat of individuality . . . that caused the word *death* to be replaced by trite circumlocutions such as 'he gave up the ghost' or 'God has his soul' "[28] was one variation on a larger discursive structure in whose terms we once knew death as something that would come purposefully to us from somewhere outside the world. There was more than one discourse that identified death as that whose purpose was to continue life in a different register. In such discourses "the fact that life has an end is not overlooked, but this end never coincides with physical death. It depends on the unknown state of the beyond, the solidity or the ephemerality of survival, the persistence of memory, the erosion of fame, and the intervention of supernatural beings. Between the moment of death and the end of survival there is an interval that Christianity, like other religions of salvation, has extended to eternity. But in the popular mind the idea of infinite immortality is less important than the idea of an extension."[29]

In fact, the sixteenth through the nineteenth centuries saw a series of discursive forms that identified in essentially erotic terms the register of a continued life beyond physical death. The life

beyond fulfilled the purposes of death's coming. Erotic represen-
tations of death ranged from the "violent" figures of the *danse
macabre* in the sixteenth century,[30] through the figures of "mystical
ecstacies of love and death . . . holy virgins dying of love, and the
little death of sexual pleasure . . . confounded with the final death
of the body"[31] of the eighteenth century. Erotic representation
changed to the still familiar figures of the romantic death in the
nineteenth century where the death of another signals "the lure of
the infinite" and "the reunion, in a beyond that is not necessarily
paradise, of all those who loved each other on earth, so that they
may prolong their early affections for eternity."[32] These forms of
discourse, from Christian to Romantic, had one thing in common:
death, though it could not be seen, was purposive and came into
the world to fulfill its purpose. All the forms of discourse that
identified death in those terms conferred on the dying person a
particular identity: the dying person was meeting the purposes of
death. This was how the dying knew himself and how others were
to know him as well.

For centuries, until the time we recognize as the origin of our
modernity, dying not only was visible but *had to be* visible. "The
dying man's bedchamber," Ariès says, "became a public place to
be entered freely. At the end of the eighteenth century, doctors
who were discovering the first principles of hygiene complained
about the overcrowded bedrooms of the dying. In the early nineteenth century, passers-by who met the priest bearing the last sacrament still formed a little procession and accompanied him into
the sickroom. It was essential that parents, friends, and neighbors
were present. Children were brought in. . . ."[33]

Whatever commanded death was totally beyond the reach of
anyone's command. Death, a wild thing that waited outside the
world and entered in its own good time, was, however, tamed by
ceremonies "both Christian and customary."[34] The ceremonies were
"organized by the dying person himself who presided over [them]
and knew [their] protocol."[35] Death's summons was a *speculum
mortes:* the mirror in which "each man would discover the secret

of his individuality''[36] and at the same time individuality's absolute limits. The wildness of death was tamed by the good fortune of being alerted to the signs of its coming and being able to prepare for the event.

This was exemplified by the "treatises on the technique of dying well, the *artes moriendi*''[37] of the fifteenth century. They stand as a paradigm of all the discursive forms that identified death and the dying until the nineteenth century. In the iconography of these treatises, liberally illustrated for the instruction of those who did not read, "the bedroom [of the dying] was to take on new meaning. . . ." It was no longer the scene of an event that was almost commonplace although more solemn than others. It became the arena of a drama in which "the fate of the dying man was decided for the last time, in which his whole life and all his passions and attachments were called into question.''[38] Heaven and hell "are present at this final ordeal that is being given to the dying man, an ordeal whose outcome will determine the meaning of his whole life. The supernatural beings are there simply as spectators and witnesses. But in that instant the dying man has the power to win or lose everything. . . . It is up to him to triumph. . . .''[39] It is worth noting that the custom of making a death mask arose because men "felt responsible for the expression their face would show in death.''[40] In other words, the death mask was like a public record of the character men showed in meeting the purpose of death.

To all of this the doctor was, at best, marginal. "Neither priest nor doctor was expected to assist the poor man in typical fifteenth— and sixteenth—century death. . . . The question whether medicine even could 'prolong' life was heatedly disputed. . . .''[41] What we cannot imagine today was reality for centuries, namely, that little if anything about dying fell under the medical aegis. When Don Juan, the Yaqui sorcerer, instructs Carlos Castaneda to look quickly so that he might see his own death just over his left shoulder where it always is,[42] he is speaking a dead language, the prose of intriguing fiction. Don Juan is speaking a language that touches an ancestral chord, but which has no basis in today's understanding of death and dying. Today we cannot think about death except in a language informed by medicine. Once it was a stroke of good fortune to be able to say to others, including the doctor if one was present at the time, "I am dying." They might respond by hoping that I was wrong and almost certainly by offering a prayer for me, but probably with little else. It would be extraordinary, today, even to hear those words spoken by the dying. If we heard them, though, our response would be instantaneous and like a reflex: "No, you're not," or, in elaborated form, "Who told you? Did the doctor tell you that?" For centuries such a response was as unthinkable as its absence is unthinkable today.

Lofland has pointed out that every social group must have rules that enable it to distinguish between the living and the dying.[43] The rules today, which are exhausted by the diagnostic signs of medicine, extend the category of the dying much farther from the actual moment of death than ever before. What is more significant, however, is that today medicine adjudicates admission to the category of the dying. Once it was the dying person himself who exclusively admitted himself to the category of the dying. It was he who warned us that he was dying. The warning, Ariès points out, "came through natural signs or, even more frequently, through an inner conviction rather than through a supernatural, magical premonition. . . . In the seventeenth century, mad though he was, Don Quixote made no attempt to flee from death into the daydreams in which he had passed his life. On the contrary, the warning signs of death brought him back to his senses: 'Niece,' he said very calmly, 'I feel that death is near.' "[44] For centuries men cut through their daydreams with these words, or words just like them. If anything separated physicians and patients it was not a privileged medical language that signified the reality of death. It was the words of the dying, speaking a common language, which invoked the reality of death. The dying spoke the words that brought to life the ceremonies and rituals that prepared them for a death that had always been expected and had now at last decided to come.

In our time we have lost the experience of death as something that comes purposefully from outside the world. We have lost the sense of death summoning us to a threshold, the other side of which is unknown but for which the dying must prepare. If this sense exists at all, it exists as an aberrant memory or a poetry that serves as counterpoint to the modern reality of death.

"After the second half of the nineteenth century," Ariès reports, "an essential change occurred in the relationship between the dying man and his entourage."[45] The dying became unwilling to know that they were dying and others became unwilling to tell them. The discourse on dying became filled with the silences, the circumlocutions and lies that denied death. The dying person assumed the identity of the patient. This capped what Ackerknecht characterizes as a "medical interest in death [that] grew all of a sudden to unique and extraordinary proportions"[46] in the eighteenth century. Concomitantly, death fell under the taboo of silence imposed on things too disgusting and revolting to speak about.[47]

The taboo on death, as all taboos must, causes us to experience what it suppresses as something wild and menacing. In this respect, the confused, alarming, painful experiences of Ivan Ilyich represent everyone's experience of death, whether they are a dying patient or not.

The idea that "death turned wild" is more than a figure of speech. It captures the general orientation toward death of people in the late eighteenth century. Then, "the problem of apparent death became abundant."[48] On the one hand humane societies "spread with an intensity comparable, perhaps, only to that of the wave of foundings of the Holy Ghost Hospitals during the twelfth century. The goal of the humane societies was to save persons drowned, asphyxiated, stricken by lightning, etc., and therefore easily confused with dead people."[49] The underside of this movement was the epidemic spread of a hysterical fear that one would be declared dead and buried alive. "Apparent death became a secularized hell."[50] In response to this terror, a virtual competition, commercial and medical-scientific, arose to find a way to discriminate between real death and apparent death. Trumpets were blown in the ears of the dead and electricity was passed through bodies.[51] Prizes were awarded for the discovery that one could detect an apparent death by detecting a faint heart beat or for suggesting "that putrefaction was the only sure sign of death" and that, therefore, the body should be kept in a mortuary to putrefy before being buried.[52] Fortunes were made on inventions of inexpensive devices that put a bell above the grave that was attached by a string to a finger of the body in the casket so that a signal could be sent in the event someone was buried alive.[53] The epidemic of fear had submerged by the late nineteenth century, but it never really disappeared. The fear of premature burial has recently resurfaced in a modern form as the fear that one might not be dead when one's organs are removed for transplanting into someone else.[54]

How, though, can a fear of being declared dead prematurely ever disappear? With the advent of modern medicine the relationship between a person and his or her own death became an alienated relationship. When medicine made death visible, it simultaneously excluded the dying person from seeing his or her own death. The iconography of the *artes moriendi,* where only the dying person and no one else could see what was transpiring in his dying, has been turned completely on its head. With the advent of modern medicine, the dying person was relegated to living his dying in the presence of the doctor who could see all.

Ivan Ilyich became possible under the rule of the great passion that the surgeon-author Richard Selzer seeks when he writes: "I have come to believe that it is the flesh alone that counts. The rest is that with which we distract ourselves when we are not hungry or cold, in pain or ecstasy. In the recesses of the body, I search for the philosopher's stone. I know it is there, hidden in the deepest, dampest cul-de-sac. It awaits discovery. To find it would be like the harnessing of fire. It would illuminate the world."[55] But medicine would only illuminate the world by plunging Ivan Ilyich into the darkness of a silence that alienates him from his own dying, that subtracts him from the body he lives and experiences.

Over the past three decades or so, things have been changing.

We are able to replace Ivan Ilyich, the paradigmatic patient, with a more defiant figure. He is clearly not as important in a literary sense but he is extremely important in a sociological sense. Ken Harrison, the principal character in Brian Clark's play *Whose Life Is It Anyway?*[56] is ninety percent the perfect patient. From the neck down his body has been rendered immobile, literally severed from his seat of consciousness, by an automobile accident that injured his spine. From the neck down, Ken is the ideal, almost pristine object of medical interest. The doctors in the play pride themselves on the work they did to save Ken from a premature death. For six months, the audience is told, medicine committed itself utterly to the restoration of Ken's bodily functions. As the play opens, Ken is almost stabilized and the staff is just about ready to discharge him to a long-term care facility where physicians and nurses will sustain Ken's bodily functions, insensible to him, for the rest of Ken's life.

But there is a problem. Ken is ten percent problem patient. He is alert, intelligent and witty. Although he is immobile, Ken can speak his mind, and he breaks the rule of silence under which medicine traditionally placed its patients by asking *the* question, whose life is it anyway? The subjective, experiential self surges forward to assert a claim over the definition of life. Medicine's hegemony over speaking true about what constitutes the patient's life is broken. But medicine resists. A junior registrar, Dr. Scott, comes to see Ken early in the play and finds him wise-cracking and almost playful. When Dr. Scott notes his demeanor, Ken wryly says something about the "courage of the human spirit." Dr. Scott, in a coolly professional manner, indifferent to any reference to the invisible except as poetic imagery, takes out her stethoscope and says, "Nice to hear the human spirit's OK. How's the lungs?" When she listens to his chest Ken, sings out a resounding "Boom. Boom." to which Dr. Scott responds, "Be quiet. You'll deafen me." Any sound, meaningful or not, will impede what auscultation is about: seeing past the patient into the body. Ken's spirit will not be silenced by Dr. Scott's way of seeing into his chest, though. In fact, Ken insists on shouting out, asserting his presence in a room quieted by the powerful gaze of the physician. He will speak, and in speaking he will deafen Dr. Scott and make a strictly medical inquiry impossible.

But the point of the play is that when Ken speaks, it is not only to discomfort medicine but to insert a new reason between the lines of medical reason. Ken Harrison decided that he wanted to be discharged from the hospital knowing full well that he would die from the buildup of his body's waste within a week of his urinary catheter being removed. The staff, naturally, refused to honor his wishes. Ken Harrison sued to seize control of his life and won. The court awarded him his life, or perhaps put more appropriately in this case, the court awarded him his death. If a play even could have been written prior to World War II that asked of medicine the question "Whose life is it?" it is unlikely the author could have arrived at the same answer.

We are in the midst of an escalating debate over the manner of our dying. The debate is rightly characterized as a social movement rather than simply the concern of intellectuals, although it is not clear how widespread the movement is. Nevertheless, we seem to have an insatiable need to talk about what it means to die and to confront the medical discourse on death with ourselves as experiencing persons. The need is not restricted to the problem of dying. Almost everywhere the experiencing person is vigorously challenging the medical discourse which subtracts him from his body. It is as if patients were bringing a scandal to light and clearing the air.

A pseudonymous patient, Anne Stewart, reports the following incident that occurred as she was recovering from a concussion: "After a night of hallucinatory fantasy, I asked my intern if this sort of manifestation was normal with respect to my injury. When he first asked to hear of my latest vision I was extremely embarrassed to relate such inanity to this little known and scientific person. After hearing my account, he told me it was a dream, that I had really been asleep and not awake as I had thought. To me, this explanation was not helpful, since the hallucinations, whether they occurred while I was awake or sleeping, continued to be a disturbing mystery."[57]

The scenario is commonplace. The patient is embarrassed over whether she should bother her doctor with certain subjective experiences. The doctor, who at least asked what happened in this case, discounts her experience as unreal. The hallucination is not normal or abnormal, as the patient's question asked; it simply was not. Finally, after being told that, in truth, she was asleep dreaming, not awake as she thought, the patient is left with a form of pain and suffering whose reality she cannot question even though the doctor may dismiss it so easily. Yet, with distinct understatement, Stewart describes her pain and suffering as "a disturbing mystery," and refuses to allow her experience to be discounted. She is more than someone who must simply listen to another who speaks true.

Chad Calland, a physician suffering from end stage renal disease who later committed suicide, provides a richer view of the new language of pain and suffering that seeks admittance to medical discourse. He wrote in the *New England Journal of Medicine*:

> Patients on dialysis are accustomed to being told by the doctor, "You are doing fine"—usually after the latest measurements of electrolytes and creatinine. The patient then thinks to himself, "If I'm doing fine, why do I feel so rotten?" After undergoing correction of several days' accumulation of metabolites in a few hours, who could feel well with the resultant cerebral edema? Who, with a hematocrit [red blood cell concentration] of 17 per cent, feels well enough to function when he cannot climb his own stairway because of dyspnea [shortness of breath]?
>
> After a number of such visits to the doctor, the patient begins to think that perhaps his very real symptoms of fatigue, dyspnea, muscle weakness and so forth are products of a deranged mind, so that he begins to conceal them because he is ashamed. Eventually, the time comes when the patient complains of nothing, and the doctor is

thus wholly unaware of these symptoms, just as he is unaware of the other (marital, financial and social) difficulties that the patient is experiencing.[58]

Calland is insisting that the medical truth of his pain and suffering is not exhausted by a language that describes the visible violence undergone by organs invaded by disease. His pain and suffering have their locus in the disruption of his body's orientation to the most fundamental and banal arrangements of things in the world. How far *up* stairs is the toilet? How far *down* is my bank account? How *near* is my wife? How *far* is the wood pile? Pain as Calland experienced it is not located in visible things within the body, nor does his pain exist in a one-to-one correspondence with his disease. Calland insists that the truth of his pain and suffering be medically acknowledged to lie in the invisible relations between his body and things outside it that medicine regards as irrelevant.

Calland's language is not a specialized, distilled, rarified, professionally limited language as is medicine's own language of pain and suffering. His is a language that seeks to bring what was once excluded and "unspoken into the order of things that are counted" where they "have a right to . . . forms of reality."[59] The "order of things" to which this new language makes reference is, simply, life itself. Medicine's own language of pain and suffering referred to diseases as entities occurring in the body, and as medicine fought against disease to eliminate the associated pain and suffering it spoke in terms of the *possibility* of life, life called into question by disease. The new language of pain and suffering speaks about *life,* not just the possibility of it. Calland, for example, speaks of life as he speaks of the pain and suffering of fellow dialysis patients: "A young woman wonders whether anyone will ever marry her, or whether she should even consider marriage. A young husband wonders whether he can, or even should, sire children and, if he does, who will support them. Older, more established patients on dialysis wonder if the struggle to live is worth the effort and money that must be put forth for the rest of their lives. Patients with growing children wonder whether these children's lives would be more damaged by continuing hemodialysis or by 'accidental' unplugging of the shunt so that at least their family's future would be more financially secure."[60] David J. Peters, a physician who was soon to die of cancer, said, "dying of cancer really doesn't take much skill—it's easy. But sometimes it's pretty hard to learn to live with cancer . . . life . . . that's the hard part."[61] Whatever else is involved in the pain and suffering imposed by disease, what is critical for the patient, according to Peters, is "a loss of control of his life."[62]

In the same vein, a story told by a member of a cancer support group reads as a story about life, not as a story about death or about cancer: "Another member had planned a large dinner party, and on the very morning of the event had learned from her physician that her cancer had metastasized. Her chief concern at that point was less a fear of death than of isolation and abandonment. She feared that her illness would evoke so much pain that she would respond to it in such a primitive, animalistic fashion that she would be shunned by others. She held her party and kept her illness secret from friends. It was with much relief that she was able to discuss these concerns in the group and to hear how other members with more advanced disease had experienced and dealt with pain."[63]

These anecdotes simply document what is becoming commonplace. In medicine the taboo on death, which represents the taboo on paying attention to the patient as an experiencing person, is being lifted. What are we to make of this? The terms in which we are to understand this lifting of the taboo are not self-evident. The image of Ivan Ilyich is fading and being replaced by patients of all sorts who will not suffer indignities to their person in silence. But, in a sense, this only sharpens the question of what is changing. Ivan Ilyich experienced the truth of the pain he suffered in the concrete terms of his existence and not just as sensations of a diseased body whose truth he could not know. These are the same thoughts patients today have. Ivan Ilyich wanted to speak them. The taboo on death caused him to experience death as wild and therefore caused him to want to speak. It caused him to want to refuse to be an object in nature. He could not become a part of that nature of which Bertrand Russell in 1909 wrote, "blind to good and evil, reckless of destruction, omnipotent matter rolls on its relentless way."[64]

Ivan Ilyich wanted to speak, but he could not because no one would take him seriously. Medical reason lay like a blanket over everyone. If Ilyich spoke it could only be the expression of painfully private emotions. It would be like giving out a great wordless cry which had no objective status because there was nothing to do about it. His speech could not be used to produce anything and therefore it belonged to the realm of the ephemeral like the subjective expression of poetic or musical sounds. It is better not to cry ugly and nightmarish sounds than to see the faces of those who have to hear them. Ivan Ilyich's wife "knows, but she does not know that he knows." As Ariès notes, "These two people might now come together in a shared truth. But Ivan Ilyich no longer has the strength to climb over the wall that he himself has built with the complicity of his family and doctors." He does not speak of what is torturing him but thinks only "What's the use of telling her? She wouldn't understand."[65] The only person in his life to whom he can eventually speak is his old servant, Gerasim. For Gerasim, who was not a modern man, dying had nothing to do with being a patient. It had everything to do with being a person and one spoke with persons even when one did not speak with patients.

We must begin to put the changes in today's patients into perspective. The question, for example, is not whether they are demanding an end to dying as patients. The demand for dignity in dying is not an attempt to move the truth of death out of the medical discourse. No one seriously claims that the "death and dying" movement is the cutting edge for a radical social change that will restore a religious society, in the serious sense of that term. The question we must ask if we wish to understand changes in today's patients is: "What *makes it possible* for them to speak today and not yesterday?" This question puts into relief what is easily missed if one is seduced by the rhetoric that describes changes in contemporary medicine as a "patient rebellion." It is less the patient who is forcing medicine to take him seriously than it is profound changes in the medical logic that governs truth-speaking. Such radical changes have occurred in medicine in the last thirty years or so that we should think of ourselves as living through a new medical revolution. The revolution is as significant as the revolution that brought modern medicine into existence around 1800. Medicine has been undergoing a transition in the structure of its discourse that not only allows the patient to speak as an experiencing person, but *needs, demands,* and *incites* him to speak.

The new medical revolution began around 1950. A prominent sign was the appearance in that year of a new text organized around the idea that the patient is a person. *Harrison's Principles of Internal Medicine,* an influential text now in its ninth edition, ushered in a new era by saying "the art of medicine is not confined to organic disease; it deals also with the mind of the patient and with his behavior as a thinking, feeling human being."[66] The content of the medical discourse was being enlarged. Instruction in identifying signs and symptoms which revealed the disease as it resided in the body would never again be sufficient preparation for the physician since, as Tinsley Harrison said in his book, mastery of the skills required in the medical encounter "depend not simply on instruction, but on emotional maturity, manifested by sensitive self-cultivation of the ability to see deeply and accurately the problems of another human being."[67] The new physician had to be able to see beyond the organs and cells accessible to the surgeon and into the unmapped depths of the human personality.

The meaning of the concepts that structure medical practice—doctor, patient, disease—were changing. The doctor-patient relationship was becoming more collegial. The implicit goal of medical care—health and cure—was being thrown up for negotiation and the doctor's search for order was no longer directed simply toward the proper operation and integration of bodily processes. The doctor's workspace was being called upon to accommodate not just disease and death, but "dying," not just women in labor and new-borns, but "birthing." Methods of monitoring patients throughout the life cycle, from conception to death, replaced technologies of invasion and correction which had characterized traditional medicine. Doctors and doctoring were reorganized around the team concept, and the doctor, like patients, became "a *human* instrument, subject to error due to the events in his own biography."[68]

The momentum generated by this transition over the past thirty years is unmistakable. In 1952, for example, Pinner and Miller introduced their book *When Doctors are Patients* by stating: "This volume is presented in the hope that the method of inquiry will be useful in defining with greater precision, to a profounder plane, and within wider limits, the *subjective experience of disease,* and, therewith, a broader field for therapeutic activities. If this particular approach be judged valid, it should undoubtedly be systematized and expanded."[69] Their language is important. In an uneffusive way Pinner and Miller are submitting the variable "subjective experience" for final judgment by the scientific authority of medicine. Two decades later Grene prefaced a similar work, *Sick Doctors,* by observing, "during a recent illness it became clear to me that the descriptions of the symptoms in medical 'literature' were very inadequate. . . . The descriptions were 'hearsay' only, second hand or worse."[70] Unlike Pinner and Miller, Grene was not submitting the efficacy of "subjectivity" for scientific, medical judgment. Grene was using it as a standard by which to judge scientific medicine, and he finds medicine wanting. Grene's call to medicine to collect "first hand" evidence of symptoms is a call back to the bedside of the speaking patient from which Bichat removed the doctor in the name of modernizing medicine. So pervasive had this view become that by 1980 it can be openly stated to the press by no less (but no more) than a third year medical student at the University of California at San Francisco: "We have already placed science on a false pedestal. . . . Biology doesn't tell the doctor how individuals will react—what their environment is, what their social background has been, what has made them sick, what will make them well."[71] By

1980, this would-be physician could state in such uneqivocal terms
what Michael Balint had said in a more circumspect way in 1957:
"It was not only the bottle of medicine or the box of pills that
mattered, but the way the doctor gives them to his patient—in fact,
the whole atmosphere in which the drug was given and taken."
Nevertheless, "no guidance whatsoever is contained in any textbook as to the dosage in which the doctor should prescribe himself,
in what form, how frequently, what his curative and his maintenance dosages should be, and so on."[72] Balint used a strained,
medically acceptable metaphor; the medical student could be less
circumspect. Their messages are the same.

It is rapidly becoming impossible for obstetricians to say, as did
Joseph B. DeLee when he entered the delivery room and noted the
contractions of labor, that they are literally seeing pain as if it
existed in one-to-one correspondence with misshapen organs caused
by pregnancy and delivery.[73] Now the obstetrician must recognize
that "cultural experience and physical environments are . . . important aspects of the childbearing experience."[74] Likewise, the
physician is called upon to be sensitive to the cultural milieu in
which a person dies. The physician is being called out from behind
his mask of power. He must speak to the woman in labor and to
the dying person, listen to their concerns, engage them in dialogue.
The new language of pain and suffering touches them both and
connects them by common experiences. It evokes a new therapeutic alliance.

Ironically, the new therapeutic alliance dissolves the physician
into a new obscurity. He becomes part of a team of people—including the patient and the patient's family. The physician is part
of a "pool of skills."[75] We are no longer to think about being born
into the hands of the doctor, but into a system of buoyancy that
supports us.

The new language of medicine is summoning forth a new definition of medical practice and is reformulating the field of medical
power. It provides new perspectives and postures, new prescriptions and proscriptions, new choices. The language is invoking the

presence of the patient, calling him forward from the far side of what once appeared to be an unbridgeable gulf. It is ending the rule of silence. No longer is medical practice to confine itself to mobilizing all its resources against pain and suffering contained and visible in the body. Now, in a way that is not yet textbook clear, medical practice is called upon to disperse itself across the network of relationships between the patient and everything else.

We must not forget that what excites us all is how Kübler-Ross got the dying to speak. But in our excitement we must not forget to try to understand what is going on. The new medical revolution has given us new experts, and first among them are the "new masters of the art of dying." They are people fashioned in the image of Kübler-Ross's students who live, in Ariès's terms, "behind a one-way mirror . . . able to observe dying persons who have agreed to talk about themselves with men of feeling and science."[76] Feeling and science are now fused in a single person: a "new master."

On one level, Kübler-Ross has restaged the anatomy lesson by placing the patient, now reconstituted as an experiencing person, under the rule of the gaze. But on another level, this restaging replaces the logo of the anatomy lesson. Until we understand the new status of the patient as an experiencing person—a status conferred by a new logic of medicine—we cannot fully understand the contemporary changes being undergone by the structure of medical power. And we cannot fully understand the new image being painted over the figures who pressed around Vesalius's dissecting table.

# Four

# Medicine's Subjective Object

D R. MICHELLE HARRISON, in her recent memoir of her medical residency in obstetrics and gynecology, raised once again the criticism that medicine treats people as objects.[1] This commonplace critique of medicine does not carry much analytical power. Indeed, once we understand that scientific medicine based its work on indifference, not hostility, toward the patient, this criticism loses much of its rhetorical power. A more valuable critical analysis of medicine derives from the fact that medicine has changed its understanding of what kind of object the patient is. The object medicine practices on today is different from the object nineteenth and early twentieth century medical doctors practiced on. Medicine practices on a subjective object, and subjectivity has been captured by medicine's new mode of objectification.

Medicine used to practice on disease. The first edition of William Osler's *Principles and Practice of Medicine,* published in 1892, did not begin with a description of the differential diagnosis or with the responsibilities of the physician; it began with a section on infectious disease, then presented sections on diseases of various organ systems, and ended with a section on diseases caused by animal parasites. This great medical text was simply a catalog of diseases. Disease was, as Leriche said it had to be, dehumanized. No people appeared in Osler's medical universe. The patient was simply a vehicle for conveying the object of medicine's attention— disease—to the workspace of the physician.

Around the middle of the twentieth century the object of medicine's attention changed. The patient's subjective experience of disease became an integral part of the object medicine practiced on. This change is marked by the replacement in medical practice of the "anomaly" by the "chronic patient" and by the merging of two discourses on life—the medical discourse concerned principally with curing disease and the socio-moral discourse concerned principally with extending compassion to the person living with a disease—that were separate but parallel during the nineteenth century. We can appreciate these changes by tracing changes in medical texts' treatments of alcoholism and pain—two problems that have always been stress points in medicine's attempts to decide how to act toward patients—and by a review of two instructive cases from the nineteenth century.

Alcoholism raises in an especially severe way for medicine the question, "What is to be done?"

The early editions of Osler's text described alcoholism by enumerating the effects of ingesting alcohol on the structures and functions of the body. Alcohol was a "poison" that caused changes in the epithelium, nerves, blood vessels and oxygen metabolism and that manifested itself "in muscular incoordination, mental disturbance, and, finally, narcosis. . . ."[2] It had "functional" effects in that it changed one's temper and "moral character" and might lead to "dementia paralytica."[3] Alcoholism could be acute or chronic, but "chronic" implied nothing more than simply a disease of long duration and poor prognosis. Osler made the distinction in his description of the treatment of alcoholism: "Acute alcoholism rarely requires any special measures, as the patient sleeps off the effects of the debauch. . . . Chronic alcoholism is a condition very difficult to treat, and once fully established the habit is rarely abandoned. The most obstinate cases are those with marked hereditary tendency. Withdrawal of the alcohol is the first essential [and is best effected through institutionalization]. . . . The absence of temptation in institution life is of special advantage. . . . Prolonged seclusion in a suitable institution is in reality the only effectual means of cure. When the hereditary tendency is strongly developed a lapse into the drinking habits is almost inevitable."[4]

While Osler describes drinking as a habit, the alcoholic is understood to be suffering from an accident. Many of them, according to this passage, suffer from a genetic accident. Medicine established the limits of its practice of discourse by suggesting that the only response to the alcoholic was social protection from the effects of his accident. The alcoholic could not be medically cured; he could only be cared for.

Little changed in this text's treatment of alcoholism during the next 50 years except the specifics of the disease. Slight adjustments in alcoholism's effects were made so that instead of causing "dementia paralytica," alcoholism was related for a while to "insanity"[5] and later to "psychoses" and a transient form of epilepsy.[6] The social problems caused by alcoholism were considered in passing by doctors.[7] Still, the only medical response to alcoholism remained institutionalization or, if a person was "fighting drunk," an "injection of apomorphine (gr. $\frac{1}{10}$, gm. 0.006) will transform the most pugnacious into a limp and docile object."[8]

Medicine spoke no truth about the alcoholic's "lived body," but only about the body as an object within which the processes of disease could be mapped. To act on the lives others lived rather than strictly on the bodies they occupied would be to exceed the limits of the truth medicine was privileged to speak. What fell outside the limits of the medical discourse was any socio-emotional expression of pain from a person whose life suffered the chronic limitation of a genetic accident. In fact, a person's pain stood outside medical discourse until very recently.

Prior to the mid-twentieth century, pain occupied little space in medical texts. It had no separate entry in Osler's indexes, much less a section of its own in his text. Pain existed in a one-to-one relationship with diseases that worked their ways through various structures in the body. Dr. Karl M. Vogel translated a turn-of-the-century German text on pain and introduced it to the "general practitioner, who is so often called upon to interpret the subjective complaint in terms of the temperament and individuality of the patient'' this way: ''In fulfilling his task the author has throughout tempered his deductions from actual pathological processes with a careful critical consideration of the functional elements which, in the phenomena of pain, so frequently cloud the clinical picture. Wherever possible, however, he has based his conclusions upon the more exact factors of anatomical structure and pathological change.''[9] The ''functional'' modification of pain which ''clouded'' the picture referred not to the effects of the emotions or to a person's social situation but to the effects of position, movement, pressure, food, drugs, and ''organic function'' on pain.[10] The book was organized much like Osler's text. It took up each organ system and outlined the various kinds of pain that might arise from each site. The patient experiencing pain did not enter into consideration.

In the 1920s pain was still an ''interpretation of some abnormal and generally harmful process which is occurring in the organism''[11] but it could be either objective or subjective. Objective pain was ''always . . . the result of some demonstrable pathological change.''[12] Subjective pains were ''those which have no physical cause for existence, but are a product of mental action arising from some changes of the coordinating centers of the sensorium.''[13] Even subjective pains had no subject attached to them. Instead they were related in a one-to-one fashion to changes in structures and could be expressed only in the disease-oriented metaphors of the day.

Nineteenth and early twentieth century doctors did not do nothing for their patients even though their logic mandated medical indifference to the patient. Doctors were, in fact, expected to feel compassion toward people whose anomalous bodies fell under their gaze. The person, besides being a collection of anatomical structures and physiological processes, was also a socio-emotional being that called forth moral, compassionate responses from others. The medical man, like others of lofty social position, was expected to be a man of compassion. It was a matter of character. Medicine accorded its practitioners a dual status. The profession provided its members an isolation and protection similar to that which the

monastery provides its monks,[14] but medicine also placed its practitioners in a high social status or simply reinforced the high social
position from which its members came. They were subject to a
moral imperative that accompanied their position and that stood
side by side with medical responsibility.

We must be clear on this point. The medical discourse only assessed the nature and extent of an accident, the "body's involvement" in a disease. A parallel but separate socio-moral practice of
compassion provided the protective response to people unfortunate
enough to suffer an accident. Compassion sought to locate individuals properly in the social order to protect victims from the
effects of their accidents. Medicine itself was not concerned with
the proper location, the "true place," of the individual even though
the agent of compassion was sometimes a medical doctor.

That the medical and socio-moral discourses were, in fact, separate is illustrated by the case of Herculine Barbin, a nineteenth
century hermaphrodite who was also known as Alexina. Alexina
was raised as a woman. She taught in a girls' school, and there she
fell in love with another teacher she calls Sara. Her life became
painful, even though it was filled with joy. When she decided to
do something about her situation she sought out a monk to hear
her confession. After two days of reflection the monk made the
ineffectual, and to Alexina, unacceptable, recommendation that she
live out her days hidden as a nun. Later a doctor was called to
examine Alexina because of pains in her groin. After an examination that left this doctor "in a state of terrible shock,"[15] he apparently explained the matter to the headmistress of the school
where Alexina worked. For reasons never made clear to Alexina
the headmistress forbade the doctor from ever entering the house
again. When the compassionate response of the monk was separated by circumstance from the medical assessments of the doctor,
neither could speak the whole truth about Alexina's situation and
neither could mobilize effective action.

Things changed when Alexina took her case to Monseigneur J.-F.

Landriot, the Bishop of La Rochelle. He listened to Alexina's confession "with a religious astonishment."[16] The bishop looked upon her with great compassion and said, "My poor child, . . . I don't yet know how all this will turn out. . . . Although I know what to think in regard to yourself, I cannot be a judge in such a matter. I shall see my doctor this very day."[17] The bishop could not know the truth fully without a medical examination. The doctor thoroughly examined Alexina and, because he alone could not decide action, he took the case back to the bishop.[18] Landriot told Alexina to return to the school and make arrangements to leave as soon as possible. His words to her were, "Have yourself replaced as soon as possible and come back here, after which we shall think about the way to make a new place for you in society."[19]

We begin to understand the nature of the compassionate response that had to be coordinated with medical inquiry in order to protect the anomaly from her accident's effects. The socio-moral discourse on life that paralleled the medical discourse on life did not call forth the emotion-laden compassion suggested by the *Oxford English Dictionary,* "the feeling or emotion, when a person is moved by the suffering or distress of another, and by the desire to relieve it."[20] The socio-moral discourse whose agent was a bishop in Alexina's case deploys a *program of compassion* whose principal purpose is to find for a person a proper place in society or, in the words of a medical doctor who examined Alexina, to find "his true place in society."[21]

The social response of programmatic compassion is uninformed without medicine. But on the other side, the medical response to the problem of a "true place" is premature without the studied deployment of a program of compassion. The two together effect what Foucault describes as a "relentless questioning" designed "to strip the body of its anatomical deceptions."[22] When separate, these two discourses on life were impotent; acting in concert they constituted a joint discourse on the truth of life that contained the power to cause lives—Herculine Barbin's life—to conform to their truth. The outcome of this power, in Alexina's case, was suicide. Her true place was in the tenements of Paris or on the rails. The problem was that she/he could not live in his/her true place.

Compassion belonged exclusively neither to the medical nor the social domain, but rather linked the two discourses while keeping them separate. Sometimes it functioned as a linkage within the person of the doctor himself, as in the case of Dr. Frederick Treves's response to John Merrick, the "Elephant Man."

Merrick, like Herculine Barbin, suffered from a genetic accident. Treves recognized Merrick's problem as an evolutionary regression and spoke of it as if Merrick were moving developmentally backwards. Treves described Merrick this way: "The transfiguration was not far advanced. There was still more of the man than of the beast. The fact—that it was still human—was the most repellent attribute of the creature. There was nothing about it of the pitiableness of the misshapened or the deformed, nothing of the grotesqueness of the freak, but merely the loathing insinuation of a man being changed into an animal."[23] This evolutionary decomposition still brings to mind a disease entity that has invaded and corrupted an unfortunate body. There was nothing medical to be done with Merrick except display him and, after he died, dissect him. As Treves put it himself after his first encounter with Merrick, "I made a careful examination of my visitor the result of which I embodied in a paper. I made little of the man himself."[24]

Treves was speaking, of course, as a doctor concerned with a doctor's truth. In fact, Treves did make much of the man but not as a doctor and not within the confines of the medical discourse. This is illustrated by Treves's later response to Merrick. After being released by his keeper and given a ticket to London, Merrick found his way to Treves, who deployed around Merrick a multifaceted program of compassion. First, he put Merrick in the isolation ward of the London Hospital even though hospital rules forbade the housing of incurables. Second, he enlisted the assistance of Mr. Carr Gomm in his efforts to gain a permanent set of rooms for

Merrick in the hospital. Carr Gomm agreed with Treves that "Merrick must not again be turned out into the world."[25] Treves, Carr Gomm, and later the public all responded to protect Merrick from the many effects of his accident by isolating him from view in the hospital. Treves did not stop with protection through isolation, however. He set up a program to help Merrick form social relationships, to find for him a place in society from which he was isolated. Treves's first step was carefully planned and executed: "I asked a friend of mine, a young and pretty widow, if she thought she could enter Merrick's room with a smile, wish him good morning and shake him by the hand. She said she could and did."[26] The response was greater than Treves had hoped for. Merrick cried and told Treves that this was the first woman who had shaken his hand. Treves's programmatic compassion reversed the evolutionary decomposition suffered by Merrick: "From this day the transformation of Merrick commenced and he began to change, little by little, from a hunted thing into a man. It was a wonderful change to witness and one that never ceased to fascinate me."[27]

By mid-twentieth century the socio-emotional developments that Treves spoke of as occurring inside his patient were no longer matters to enthrall the compassionate physician. They were technical concerns that were becoming central to the medical discourse. The medical discourse was expanding to become something more than strictly medical. It would merge with the socio-moral discourse and make compassion and the social aspects of medicine technical matters to be mastered by a good physician much like one mastered a surgical technique.

For example, in 1942 alcoholism acquired a psychological dimension in the eyes of medicine. While alcoholism was not included among a new class of diseases known as psychosomatic disorders, diseases that were "essentially non-organic,"[28] its treatment changed to include psychological considerations. The 14th edition of Osler's text retained its recommendation for "prolonged seclusion in a suitable institution" but it added the following qualification: "Others think a rather brief stay in an institution followed by prolonged direction by a neuropsychiatrist is more effective. For success the patient himself or herself must seek voluntarily such guidance and be convinced that an occasional drink will prevent cure."[29]

The 1947 edition of *The Principles and Practice of Medicine* added consideration of the patient's social situation to medical inquiry. It said, "In many illnesses the chief cause lies in conflicts and maladjustments developing from the patient's family and marital relationships, his associations and friendships, his economic problems, his occupation, his business, etc. It is the patient's reactions to past and present happenings of many sorts that determine or at least color many of the symptoms he complains of and which constitute his illness."[30] But social situation could only be used in diagnosis; it was not an explicit part of the problem, the illness or disease, yet. The 1968, 17th edition of Osler's text treated alcoholism as a disease of the liver and advised the doctor, "Alcoholism is suggested by a sloppy personal appearance, by failure to consult a physician until the disease has advanced far beyond a stage that would normally be alarming to people of comparable educational and social standing, and by the patient's reluctance to enter a hospital."[31] Treatment remained largely psychological and the main task of medicine remained treatment of concomitant problems such as hypoglycemia, coma, and pneumonia.

In the 1970s alcoholism acquired an explicitly social dimension. In the 1972 edition of *The Principles and Practice of Medicine,* alcoholism changed from a disease to "but one of a number of maladaptive ways of dealing with life's stresses and is best regarded as a symptom of such maladaptation. . . ."[32] Recommended treatment changed from medical isolation and protection from the effects of a genetic accident (since "no convincing underlying or predisposing genetic, physical, or metabolic abnormality has been identified despite considerable effort to do so"[33]) to programmatic compassion. Compassion, however, was now within medicine, not something that stood to the side of medical practice and acted in concert with it. The text told the physician to treat the patient "as an individual and . . . forego old stereotypes of alcoholics." Counseling designed to find the patient's proper place in a dynamic social community became the preferred approach to alcoholism: "Counseling includes exploring the patient's capacity for alternative modes of adaptation and formulating appropriate medical interventions. It is worthwhile assuming that the patient would not be alcoholic if such alternative modes were easily available and readily apparent to him; for this reason simple exhortations to 'will power' usually fail."[34] With this passage a simple psychological approach to alcoholism was abandoned and the search for non-maladaptive means of living a life became an explicit medical responsibility.

By 1980 alcoholism was no longer considered even a symptom, a term which evokes notions of underlying disease entities. It had become a "behavior disorder" characterized by either "psychological or physiological dependence on alcohol," "impairment of physical or mental health," or "impairment of the individual's functioning at home, school, work, or in any other sector of his life."[35] Alcoholism was now three-dimensional—biophysical, psychological, and sociological—and preferred treatment reflected this conceptualization. Texts recommended abstention enforced perhaps by alcohol antagonists, counseling in a clinic, and involvement of "the close members of the family in the evaluation of the patient's condition and in the development of a plan of treatment."[36] The biophysical and sociological, if not socio-moral, had been joined under a newly elaborated medical discourse.

Pain, like alcoholism, gained a socio-emotional dimension around World War II and became central to medical inquiry. Tinsley Harrison's *Principles of Internal Medicine* devoted an entire section to pain. The section immediately followed the text's introduction which instructed the physician on "The Approach to the Patient."[37] The socio-moral discourse on life joining the medical discourse on life made the subjective patient medicine's new object of inquiry and made a person's experience of pain a central aspect of the medical encounter. As Harrison put it in 1950, "The reaction of the person to pain depends in part on the meaning of the sensation interpreted in the light of past experiences. . . . Pain has a large emotional as well as purely physical component."[38] The socio-emotional aspects of pain no longer cloud the clinical picture; they are an integral part of pain, which becomes the pivot around which the entire clinical picture of the patient as a person is organized. The feeling, thinking, subjective patient—the whole person—becomes the new object of medical inquiry.

Medicine's new vision of the patient and the new importance attached to the patient's pain were but the tip of a very deep-seated, fundamental reformulation of medical work and medical power. A disease that is an entity in the body called forth a medical-curative response. The disease of long duration with poor medical prognosis—the chronic disease—called forth a compassionate, protective, social response. To medicine of the post-war era disease is much more than an entity in the body and calls forth an elaborated medical response that is more than medical. In the words of *Butterworth's Medical Dictionary* (1978): "A disease is the sum total of the reactions, physical and mental, made by a person to a noxious agent entering his body from without or arising from within. . . . Since a particular agent tends to produce a pathological and clinical picture peculiar to itself, although modified by individual variations in different patients, a mental concept of the average reactions or a composite picture can be formed which, for the convenience of description, is called a particular disease or clinical entity. But a disease has no separate existence apart from a patient, and the only entity is the patient."[39] Medicine invented the patient who was also a person, for the first time in its history, when new rules for speaking truth emerged.

The new rules of medical inquiry were organized not around the taxonomic logic and anatomical perspective of the nineteenth and early twentieth century but around a systems-theoretic logic and an ecological perspective. Mechanistic relationships in the body lost their prominence to relationships mediated by information flows in a broader ecology. The domain of the doctor expanded. The socio-moral definition of life was joined with the biophysical definition of life to form a single medical discourse on life that was something greater than the traditional, strictly confined medical discourse.

*Five*

# The New Medical Logic: Relationships, Information Flows, Systems

THE ROYAL SCOTTISH MUSEUM in Edinburgh has a remarkable collection of birds. Jammed into cases around an upper pavilion, thousands of specimens from all over the world are arranged according to genera, species, and subspecies. Only the most discerning, well-trained eye can see the differences that the specimen tags announce. A fleck of white or a slightly different beak angle, invisible to the naive observer, makes, quite literally, all the difference in the world when one must distinguish between one specimen and another. The taxonomist, after years of instruction and study, is comfortable here; the lay person is not. The less well informed are attracted to the exhibits downstairs that place many different animals in a representation of their natural ecology. The differences between animals are obvious there; but, more important, the differences acquire meaning as a result of being shown something about the relationships among animals as they occur in nature. Even in static tableaux, characteristics of birds—their color, size, the shape of their beaks, and so on—take on so much more meaning when shown in relation to lizards, animals, grasses, trees, and landscapes than they do when birds are simply displayed, stuffed, with other similar birds.

It was almost inevitable that the practices of differentiation, speciation, and instruction necessary to hone an acute, penetrating medical gaze should give way to an encompassing incorporation, a gaze that attributes meaning to a phenomenon—disease, health, birth, death—in terms of its relations to things in its ecology rather than in terms of slight differences from things most like it. A taxonomic approach to medicine which seeks to differentiate further the hyper-differentiated leads to few advances in regimes of care. As diseases are conceptually refined, treatment schemes can be also, but only rarely does the micro-surgical separation of one disease from its related kinship of diseases foster a major re-thinking of medical approaches to that family of diseases or spawn a radically new approach to care. But when the gaze places a disease in its ecology and notes all of the variables from many parts of the environment that are crucial to the very existence of that disease, a plethora of alternative approaches to "treatment" presents itself to the physician.

An ecological orientation to medicine, which entered medical discourse with force some time around 1950, changes the logic of medical inquiry. Instead of locating death and identifying disease by isolating the specific causal chain of energies and events occurring in the body, an ecological perspective locates all phenomena of interest to medicine in terms of the sometimes obvious, sometimes obscure relations to other phenomena and events in the ecology that have a bearing on the disease's coming into existence and on its mode of activity. An ecological perspective shifts attention away from mechanically or electrically juxtaposed events and toward relationships mediated by information flows in systems. The rise of ecological medicine expands the realm of medical discourse beyond the limits of the body. Specifically, the body as the patient experiences it, with all of the relationships a person has in the social world, becomes an important element in the new medical logic.

To understand the nature of the new medical logic, consider the factory. The factory is not an organization of people; it is an organization of work. To design a factory someone must analyze the process of making the desired product in order to lay bare the finest possible details of that process. Perhaps ironically, the product loses importance as one begins to design a factory to build it. It fades into the background to become a guiding vision, that on which all the disparate activity inside and outside the factory must ultimately converge, but which remains directive and invisible until the very last moment in production. The process of manufacture becomes prominent, and the process must be divided and subdivided into individually meaningless activities, each of which can be done repetitively, efficiently, and thoughtlessly by a person or a machine at the behest of the manager, the one person who knows not only the goal of everyone's work but also the tiniest segments of each activity which contribute to achieving the factory's goal.

Once the production process is finely analyzed and subdivided, the manager must consider the relationships among individual workers and machines that are most likely to produce the product well but inexpensively. The manager is not concerned principally with the interpersonal relationships among workers, but with the relationships among parts of the production process. The movement of material and the intimately known processes of production govern spatial organization.

Once the factory is organized and production begins, the manager must monitor the entire process including aspects of production external to the factory. He must insure that he receives regular information concerning supplies of raw material, worker absenteeism, the speed of production at every point in the factory, even the supply of unemployed people in the community available for work should some catastrophe strike his work force. In turn, he must send out information to every point in the plant: order more raw material, speed up work here, slow it down there, increase the file of unskilled laborers' applications. The manager, guided by a vision of a product, must first differentiate the production process, then attend to the relationships among material and personnel, create information channels that will keep the production process moving smoothly and use those information channels effectively.

Frederick Winslow Taylor developed the tools by which modern production processes could be divided up and allocated among workers. During the last part of the nineteenth century, at about the same time "regular," scientific medicine solidified its social and legal bases, Taylor formulated his method, which he called "scientific management."[1] Taylor's time and motion studies of the simplest activities—picking up a wrench, turning a bolt three-quarters of a turn, putting down a wrench—allowed managers to organize finely divided production processes efficiently. But dividing up production processes in order to control production forced managers to pay more attention to *worker* control than they ever had before because the worker who failed to do his or her task in precisely the manner prescribed by the manager fouled the entire process and kept the factory from realizing the vision around which everything was organized. The idiosyncracies of workers that arise because they are thinking, feeling, willful people had no place in the modern factory. Discipline had to replace the threat of personal quirks.

To improve worker control, managers had to look deeper and deeper into production processes. Looking deeper did not mean subdividing the process of production further; it had been subdivided to the fullest possible extent already. Looking deeper meant expanding one's scope of interest. The system of production in the factory with its inputs, outputs, processes, relationships and information flows, was, in the manager's expanded scope of interest, only one aspect of the production process. Workers' home lives, the social system of the town in which the factory was located, the economic system of the town, nation, and world, as well as workers' psychologies all impinged on the factory's production. Managers could control many relationships within the walls of the factory and make adjustments as necessary; events outside remained out of their control but they were crucial nonetheless and demanded consideration and monitoring. Businesses hired economists to assess their factory's relations to the rest of the economy, to monitor information received from the economic environment, and to write reports required by various elements of the environment such as governments. Businesses also hired public relations people to send out information deemed useful to their cause. They hired planners, architects and social workers to design "company towns" best suited to the production of their product. They employed psychologists to insure that morale remained high and that psychological troubles did not interfere with production. And they hired doctors and set up clinics to treat the sick and to certify claims of illness that caused absence from work.

The manager became a management team constantly assessing all aspects of the environment that affected production and ultimately the realization of a vision. An interdisciplinary team was necessary because a disruption at any level in the ecology of the factory could disrupt production. Conceptually the level of the factory became equal in importance to the level of the world economy on which the factory depended for its supply of raw material. To analyze, organize, monitor, and manage complicated production processes, the interdisciplinary management team turned to the antidisciplinary logic of systems theory that rescued Taylor's practices of analysis and division from their own likely burial in the well-dissected details of production processes.

Traditional, scientific medicine was built on the practices of differentiation and speciation. Differentiation and analysis occurred at many levels: at the level of diseases, at the level of diagnosis, at the level of medical practice as medicine acquired the ability to isolate parts of the body from other parts, and at the level of the organization of medicine as specialties multiplied. Differentiation continues today, and medicine still seems to thrive on the discovery of new diseases (Legionnaire's disease, or the various problems that fads bring like "aerobics ankle," for example), new techniques of intervention in disease processes (microsurgery), new diagnostic procedures (computerized axial tomography and automated scanners to do it), and the development of new subspecialties (oncology has recently spawned geriatric and pediatric oncology, for example). But the traditional approach to medicine reached a point of diminishing returns years ago.

In the early 1960s in his Silliman Lectures at Yale University, René Dubos criticized medicine for its lack of flexibility and adaptability: "The tenacity with which orthodox medical institutions are pursuing the dream of defining all the 'minute particulars' of life constitutes proof of their admirable stability. But stability without adaptability to the new problems posed by modern life is socially dangerous and perhaps suicidal." For Dubos the separation from the social realm and the isolation afforded medicine by the hospital reduced the likelihood of major medical advances: "The luxurious hospitals, lavish research facilities, and scientific programs of training, of which we are justifiably so proud, are likely to appear within a few decades as magnificent cenotaphs to concepts which once were vital forces but which are no longer generating truly new scientific departures." Medicine, Dubos suggested, would continue to prosper for many years, but it would gain only the prosperity that comes from the inertia of a fast-moving, rather ponderous body. He predicted that the disciplines of scientific medicine "will eventually founder in a sea of the irrelevant if they become hypnotized by their own self created problems, and continue to neglect those presented by real life."[2] Real life was for Dubos and is for us who live most of our lives outside medicine that vast set of interrelationships among people and things that forms the biological and social ecosphere of the earth.

We know now that Dubos was not so much a critic or a prophet when he wrote *Man Adapting* in 1965 as he was an acute interpreter of trends that had been set in motion two decades earlier. Dubos coaxed medicine down the path on which it started in 1950, a path that would lead to a new medical logic. The development of the new medical logic went through three roughly cumulative stages. First, patient psychology was accorded separate attention but was fitted into the context of total medical care. Patient psychology did not become a separate, distinct specialty but a complementary aspect of all other specialties' care. Second, the patient—his/her psychology plus anatomic structures and vital functions—was placed in an ecology, and the profession expanded the scope of its gaze to encompass the ecology as well as the patient. In effect, the physician's "patient" got bigger. Third, the profession embraced a logic that would grasp the ecology and hold it up for analysis just as the logic of the anatomist had grasped the body and held it up for analysis earlier. Medicine turned to, or more accurately, medicine is turning to the boundary-breaching logic of systems theory. A new vision of the concept of "understanding" was generated through an inversion of the old meaning of the term. Understanding was no longer understood in terms of reducing the complex to the simple; now understanding called for locating the simple in relation to the complex.

The introductory section on the physician's "Approach to the Patient" in the ninth (1980) edition of *Harrison's Principles of Internal Medicine* was an inverted form of the same section in the first (1950) edition of this text. The first edition began by emphasizing the importance of diagnosis and concluded with the complementary importance of attending to a patient's psychology; the ninth edition began with the subjective, experiential aspects of illness. "An aspect of illness that influences the physician-patient relationship is the real or implied significance of disease in the mind of the patient,"[3] the first page of the text says. Regardless of the objective truth of the disease as known to the physician's informed gaze, the new truth of disease cannot be known without entering that complementary psychological realm of the mind.

Paying attention to the patient's psychology in the post-1950 era was not just a new component of humane care—something that a physician should do because it was "nice." Physicians found that when they considered the psychological realm, new therapeutic options were opened to them. The patient's psychology was a new entree to patient control. Psychological management was often as effective as, and usually less expensive and less dangerous than, old methods of control. So, for example, as obstetrics moved away from general anesthesias and toward local anesthesias, the profession also began to be concerned with patients' environments and embraced the techniques of natural childbirth. As early as 1945, professionals worried about providing a "cheerful atmosphere" in "comfortable surroundings" and became concerned with what staff members said when they could be overheard by patients. The environment had to be controlled to improve the management of birth.[4] As early as 1952, many obstetricians recognized the value of natural childbirth techniques and chastised their colleagues for not endorsing them: "We believe that the few people who are criticizing the method have not given it a fair trial or else may have suffered a deflation of the ego when they saw how successfully a patient could accomplish, with proper preliminary training, what a physician has been trained for years to do with all sorts of specialized drugs and instruments."[5] Medicine transformed the patient's personality from something that at best was irrelevant to medical work and at worst interfered with it into something that could be used to improve medical work. The management of the subjective aspects of illness complemented the management and treatment of the traditional, objective aspects of disease.

René Dubos turned his criticism of medicine into the next step forward in the pursuit of a new medical logic. In *Man, Medicine, and Environment,* he noted first that psychology complemented traditional medical practice: "Whatever its precipitating cause and its manifestations, almost every disease involves both the body and the mind, and these two aspects are so interrelated that they cannot be separated one from the other." But in the very next sentence he located the psycho-physiological patient in its ecology and accorded almost equal emphasis to the relations between people and the environments as he had to the relations between mind and body: "The understanding and control of disease require that the mind-body complex be studied in its relations to external environment. Most immediate medical problems have their origin in the responses of the human organism to present environmental forces."[6] Dubos tried to be the model investigator for others. Instead of taxonomically pursuing the minute particulars of his own discipline, microbiology, Dubos ventured far afield, well outside his area of certified competence. He has been criticized, as he expected to be, "for lack of knowledge and errors of judgment"[7] in some areas he explored, but he remains an acknowledged pivotal figure in the history of medical thought because he offered a new way of understanding health and illness. Just as the curator brings a new, clearer meaning to birds and their minute characteristics by putting them into an ecological setting in museum tableaux, Dubos opened new vistas for medicine by insisting that "present concepts concerning the delivery of medical services, including diagnosis, therapeutic procedures, and after-care, . . . be recast to adapt them not only to present knowledge but especially to local conditions,"[8] that is, to the ecology.

Ecological medicine evolved from the strange and somewhat suspect hybrid discipline of psychosomatic medicine and entered medical school curricula in the late 1960s. As described by a faculty member of Albert Einstein College of Medicine, "Ecological medicine is more than comprehensive medicine or psychological medicine because its tasks ⟨are⟩ to recogniz⟨e⟩, evaluat⟨e⟩, prevent and treat all the physical, psychological, socioeconomic and cultural variables which are an integral part of the disease process."[9] By the late 1970s, new textbooks, especially those that sought to reintegrate fields that had drifted apart like obstetrics, neonatology, and pediatrics, almost had to begin with a section on "The *Ecology* of Patient Care."[10]

With increasing frequency in the early 1970s, articles appeared calling for a new biomedical model. In fact, most people did not want simply a new *biomedical* model because they found that term too constraining. It implied a narrow range of inquiry and a reductionist search for the ultimate causes of disease in the physico-chemical processes of the body. This was precisely what the reformers did not want. They wanted a new model that would encompass the ecology which medicine had started to include in its thinking. George Engel, for example, wanted a "biopsychosocial" model for medicine.[11] Others seemed to want a physico-chemico-bio-psycho-socio-politico-economico-ecological model. Without exception, though, those calling for a new model turned medicine's attention to systems theory because it offers a logic capable of handling multilayered conceptualizations of phenomena.

Ludwig von Bertalanffy revolutionized biological thinking in 1950 with the publication of two papers on general systems theory which he later followed with a book that summarized many of the ideas he developed through the 1930s and 1940s.[12] It seems strangely appropriate that von Bertalanffy should have judged the intellectual climate unreceptive to his ideas during the decades prior to 1950, and therefore withheld them from publication until he was encouraged to publish by an interdisciplinary group including Kenneth Boulding, an economist; J. G. Mills, a psychiatrist-psychologist; and Anatol Rapoport, a mathematician.

Von Bertalanffy's systems theory was not so much a theory as a way of thinking. Systems theory provides one with a set of concepts that helps organize one's thinking about complicated processes and about the large arrays of distantly as well as proximally related system components that produce them. Regardless of the level at which one begins to examine a complex system, processes that are similar to those occurring at other levels are evident: processes of input and output selectivity, encoding of information sent and decoding of information received, positive and negative feedback processes, memory and storage processes, and so on. Systems theory is a theory of the general processes that occur in all systems, their subsystems, and their suprasystems.

In the early 1940s, critics appeared in medicine who challenged their own profession to adopt a systems-theoretic point of view. For example, Kenneth Walker became medicine's museum curator who attributed meaning to disease by locating it carefully in an ecology when his book, *The Circle of Life,* was published in 1942. He also became one of the earliest proponents of the systems perspective. Of disease he said, "When we looked at disease from the standpoint of the individual, we were unable to find meaning in it, and we were forced to regard it as an unfortunate accident. Now that we have stood further away from our subject, and we have viewed illness on the larger scale of life on the earth, it begins to acquire a new significance,"[13] the significance a tableau-like stage provides. To step back and gain this larger-scale view, a new logic was necessary, and Walker described it in terms that are familiar today:

> Fortunately, we are witnessing a reaction from [the] departmentalized and "broken-machine" view of illness, just as we are witnessing a reaction from a mechanistic explanation of the universe. . . . Matter has now been identified with energy and the scientist has repainted the picture by which he represents the universe. For space occupied by myriads of solid atoms he has substituted a space-time continuum disturbed by vibratory differentiations. Medicine obediently follows the lead given by the scientist, and since the scientist has substituted a dynamic for a static picture of the universe, so must the doctor now substitute a dynamic for a static view of life. He can no longer regard a sick man as a broken machine, but must look upon him as being an energy system in which the balance of forces has been disturbed. An up-to-date definition of illness would, therefore, be to the effect that it is an upsetting of the equilibrium of an energy system, by the impact of some hostile force. Disease is a state of disequilibrium.[14]

Oddly, given this early urging, but perhaps understandably, given medicine's deliberate separation from the social realm and the inertia from which Dubos said medicine suffered, medicine discovered systems theory rather late. It took longer for the intellectual climate of medicine to become receptive to systems theory, and its approach to this very general, purposefully encompassing set of ideas is still painfully tentative. But in the early 1970s, some fifteen years after other disciplines started toying with systems theory, articles which offered the theory to a reluctant profession began appearing in the literature.

Howard Brody, for example, spelled out the utility and implications of systems theory for medicine in a paper published in 1973.

Brody explained how, from a systems perspective, "the individual human being is both a natural system and a hierarchy of natural systems." The figure reproduced here as Figure 5.1 represents "Man" as a hierarchy of systems in which the "Person"—which according to Brody can be only "loosely labeled" and identified— is embedded. Crucial to maintaining the hierarchy of systems is appropriate information flow between levels and between the hierarchy of systems and its environment. Systems theory makes any subset of the hierarchy equivalent to any other subset by focusing attention on the similarity of information flows and feedback loops which must occur at all levels in order to maintain the hierarchy's dynamic stability. Figure 5.2 shows how information flows can be abstracted from their specific subsystem contexts shown in Figure 5.3 and how information flows become the common denominator for thinking about the entire ecology of patient care. Interplay between the hierarchy and its environment reciprocally affects and shapes both while information flows within the hierarchy relay notices of disruptions in the hierarchy or changes in the environment and facilitate adaptive changes.[15]

Systems theory demands rethinking of basic medical concepts. It encourages one to concentrate on dynamic processes, not just the static structure, of the "Man" hierarchy. It encourages "a more phenomenological view of disease . . . concerned with the relationships among disease, personality, bodily constitution, and environment for neither organism nor environment is a static structure which can be separated, but both together are opposing directions in the total biological process." If the body thus loses its privileged place in medical thinking, so does the notion of causality and its attendant explanatory logic that the informed gaze brought to the medical encounter previously: "Organismic disease theory has been preoccupied with the role of microorganisms in producing disease. . . . Yet, even their part in producing infectious disease is a necessary rather than sufficient cause, and their mode of action is far from understood, since many normally occurring organisms may under certain conditions become pathogenic."[16] Systems theory

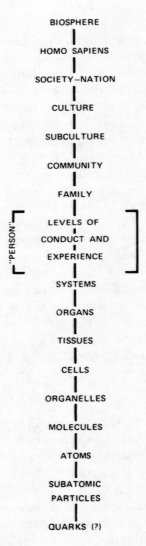

FIGURE 5.1 Hierarchy of natural systems constituting "Man." Reproduced, with permission, from Howard Brody, "The Systems View of Man: Implications for Medicine, Science, and Ethics," *Perspectives in Biology and Medicine* 17 (Autumn, 1973), p. 74. © 1973 by The University of Chicago.

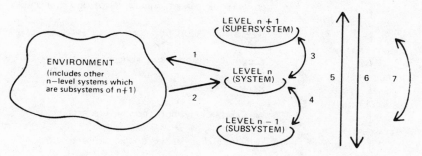

Key:

1. Manipulation: Norms of system projected onto environment

2. Adaptation: Elements of environment mapped onto system, with readjustment of system norms

3. Interlevel feedback between level n + l and level n

4. Interlevel feedback between level n and level n − l

5. Multilevel positive feedback: forces of evolution and growth by formation of new sypersystems

6. Multilevel negative feedback: control of subsystems by systems at higher hierarchical levels

7. Bypass feedback: see discussion in text under "Systems Definition of Health and Disease."

FIGURE 5.2 Summary of major types of information flow affecting level *n* in a hierarchy of natural systems. Reproduced, with permission, from Brody (see fig. 5.1), p. 76. © 1973 by The University of Chicago.

encourages the physician to look to the distant "conditions" which foster or accentuate, inhibit or attenuate the pathogenic action of a microorganism rather than paying strict attention to the proximal conditions such as the effects of organic lesions.

"Health" becomes like the product that informs the organization of the factory. It is not, in itself, important, but as a vision it is crucial. The new medical logic makes important the patient's experience of disequilibria—both those inside the body and those

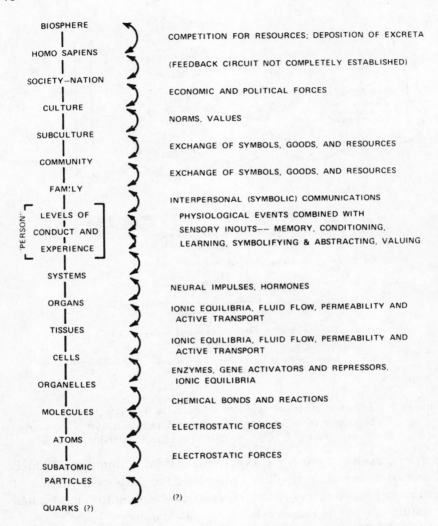

FIGURE 5.3 Nature of feedback signals at various interlevel feedback loops in the "Man" hierarchy. Reproduced, with permission, from Brody (see fig. 5.1), p. 77. © 1973 by The University of Chicago.

outside it—that are disease. The patient-physician relationship becomes ambiguous, for systems theory forces us to ask, what exactly is the "patient" in the hierarchy of systems that constitutes "Man," and what exactly does the physician "treat"? Systems theory casts a bright light on these difficult questions so troublesome to traditional medicine, which was content to look inside the body, locate the disease, and treat it there. They are questions from which medicine would like to turn, but medicine's course is irreversible. Medicine's new logic changed the parameters of the medical encounter and thereby forced medicine to confront these questions. They are the questions with which it is struggling today.

# Six

# Disease, the Doctor, and the Individual

THE DOCTOR, THE PATIENT, the disease. These are the parameters of the medical encounter. All change under the new medical logic. The notion of disease expands to include disturbances in parts of the "Man" hierarchy of systems (called the "holon") other than those parts that constitute the human being. As the notion of disease expands, so must the medical gaze. The physician must consider real, legitimate and relevant to the medical encounter aspects of life not captured by the informed gaze previously. This requires a reformation of the role of the physician. The physician must become a facilitator, a negotiator, a team member dedicated not to the treatment of disease but to the management of each patient. The patient, in turn, becomes an individual, something more than a set of physiological processes capped with a peculiar personality. An individual is the unique grounding for all disturbances in the holon, the privileged entity that gives meaning and significance to the environment. The patient was only a bearer of data, that which conveyed a disease into the field formed by the medical gaze; the individual supplies information but also stands in judgment of elements in his or her environment including medicine and the nature of care received. The individual has a voice and speaks. The physician operating under the new medical logic must do more than listen; the physician-manager must enter into a dialogue with the patient-individual and formulate strategies for managing those difficulties which the individual identifies as problematic. The physician and the patient must engage in a "joint adventure," a notion that forms a nucleus around which medical work is being reorganized.

First, consider the meaning of "disease." Like *Butterworth's Medical Dictionary,* Howard Brody identifies disease as a failure of some structure or system in the holon hierarchy of systems to conform with the overall pattern of the holon. "This state of failing to conform is generally precipitated by some disruptive force or perturbation from the external environment—here again using 'external' in the broad sense and remembering that what is external to one cell in a tissue may be internal to the tissue, and so on. These perturbations may be extremely precise in terms of which hierarchical levels they impinge upon—for example, radiation primarily affects the level of subatomic particles—or they may be very broad, as in the trauma of an automobile collision. It seems reasonable to identify the disruption of the hierarchical structure that results from such a perturbation with the concept of disease."[1]

There are two very important aspects of this definition. "Disease" is not a highly specific idea. Disease is simply a disruption somewhere in the hierarchy and the hierarchy is all-encompassing, extending literally from quarks to the biosphere. The medical gaze must become an encompassing gaze surveying all there is to be seen rather than concentrating narrowly on the identification of diseases that occur within the body. This points to the second important difference between the traditional notion of disease and the new, systemic, ecological notion of disease. The new notion locates disease in terms of patterns, structures, and relationships among components of intricately related systems, whereas the old notion required that a disease be isolated, located and identified as an entity unto itself. The anatomist-surgeon opened a body and saw diseased tissues and could reconstruct the sequence of events that produced the disease as its end state. Now disease is identical to disturbed relationships—structures that do not conform to overall system patterns—in complex, dynamic, large holons. Systems theory, the basis of the new medical logic, presents the physician with "a conceptual framework that can account for such effects as those of environment, personal and social history, or genetic make-up on individual, biological and social relationships to health and disease,"[2] quite in contrast to the old approach to medical inquiry organized around the idea "that disease is a thing in itself, essentially unrelated to the patient's personality, his bodily constitution, or his mode of life."[3]

Nineteenth century medicine "regulated in accordance with normality,"[4] excluded the anomaly and created it as an object of compassion in the fault lines that run in the interstices of societies—in the traveling freak shows, in the tenements of Paris, and as an occasional worker on the railroads. Medicine did its work in hospital, an "enclosed, pestilential domain."[5] There was no room in nineteenth century medicine or hospitals for the anomaly. Mid-twentieth century medicine made room for the anomaly by reconstituting medicine's institutional form. Medicine became an integrated organization that extended outside the boundaries of the hospital and managed patients instead of treating diseases. The organization would be regulated not in accordance with normality but in accordance with social utility and would incorporate the anomaly by creating him or her as the "chronic patient" in need of total care.

The roots of changes in medicine lie in the 1920s and 1930s when concern over the incidence of chronic diseases in non-institutional populations first surfaced. States conducted health surveys.[6] The National Health Survey of 1935 collected information on the personal, social, and economic impact of chronic disease.[7] The National Hygenic Laboratory became the National Institute of Health in 1930. In turn, the NIH developed a single categorical program in cancer prior to World War II (1937) and six other categorical programs after the war with the final two, the National Institute of Arthritis and Metabolic Disease and the National Institute of Neurological Disease and Blindness, being established in 1950.

With the National Institutes in place, federal effort devoted to chronic disease mushroomed. In 1946 the American Hospital Association, the American Medical Association, the American Public Health Association, and the American Public Welfare Association formed the Joint Committee on Chronic Disease, which published its final report, *America's Health,*[8] in 1949. In June 1949, the Commission on Chronic Illness, a direct descendant of the Joint Committee, was incorporated; it published its multi-volume report in 1957. In 1951, President Truman established the Commission on the Health Needs of the Nation, whose 1953 report[9] devoted considerable attention to chronic illness. In January 1955, the first number of the *Journal of Chronic Disease* appeared in direct response to the concerns of the President's Commission. All of these events created a rhetoric directed to the reorganization of medical care.

At the conceptual level, the problem was to locate disease in the socio-economic parts of the holon hierarchy of systems. "Chronic diseases create not only medical problems, they are a major cause of social insecurity," said Ernst Boas in 1940. "Their malign influence permeates into all phases of our living, causing indigency and unemployment, disrupting families and jeopardizing the welfare of children."[10] Chronic diseases cause disruption and disharmony in the economy: "Altogether it has been estimated that chronic disease results in half to three-quarters of a billion man-days per year lost from productivity. Chronic illness also accounts for public expenditures of about $1.5 billion a year for medical and hospital services and about $1.5 billion for cash benefits."[11] The disruptive effects propagate down and up through various layers of the social system. To the family, "chronic illness often presents an overwhelming financial problem," which reflects upwards to cause "dependency on public funds."[12]

The problem of finding a "true place," a *productive* place, for the person who used to exist outside the productive system as an anomaly creates a rationale for attaching the socio-moral definition of life directly to the biophysical definition of life to create a new medical discourse. The new discourse can speak of disease at three separate levels. Diseases or defects in the body are "impairments" which manifest themselves at the personal-behavioral level as "disabilities" which, in a social context of specific performance expectations, become "handicaps."[13] Medicine has incorporated into its work that realm of concerns previously reserved for the socioemotional discourse that centered on compassion.

In practice, this new medical discourse requires an incorporative, integrated structure in order to detect disease where it is located, in the social body. "The hospital," Foucault says, "is an artificial locus in which transplanted disease runs the risk of losing its essential identity."[14] The hospital abstracts the disease from the person who is incidental to it and who makes the disease impure. Placing the person back in the community can obscure the disease as it exists in its pure state in the body. "The majority of individuals afflicted [with chronic illness] reach a state of equilibrium, in which they live happily for many years, in spite of their disability. These people when examined by a physician usually exhibit a number of pathological findings, but their symptoms and complaints are negligible."[15] To discover chronic diseases, which Boas describes as "a hidden and insidious plague . . . all the more deadly, for its wide range is hardly recognized. . . ,"[16] medicine had to constitute itself into an integrated structure that penetrates into the social body outside the hospital. Medicine organized itself around the concept of "prevention."

Osler felt that one prevented a disease by studying its etiology and "rendering . . . conditions in the body unfavorable for its propagation and action."[17] Prevention now involves much more than Osler's enlightened and "rational" approach to the body of the patient. Prevention today requires broad-based attention to social organization.

> To bring about maximum utilzation [of knowledge and
> measures for the prevention of chronic disease] poses
> problems of professional education, of organization and

administration. How can the concept of prevention be instilled in students of medicine, nursing, social work, health education, and related disciplines? What organizational patterns will be most effective for the administration of preventive programs? How can the public be moved to adopt and support preventive measures? . . . Prevention of chronic illness and disability requires mobilization of individual and public resources, in all aspects of health protection and health care. Freedom from chronic illness can be achieved only through united efforts: (1) toward health promotion; (2) toward preventing the occurrence of illness; and (3) toward early detection of disease through health examinations and mass screening programs to assure treatment in the early stages that will prevent disability or premature death."[18]

Such a wide medical net requires that medicine be organized internally into "health care teams" which articulate with community-based screening programs. The first experiments with health care teams occurred in 1950 at the Montefiore Hospital (Bronx, New York). In 1920, Montefiore became the first hospital to orient its services specifically toward people with chronic illnesses. "This was an isolated action; it was the first time that persons suffering from chronic diseases were treated as patients needing care, not as incurable invalids."[19] As the conceptualization of chronic illness changed, so did the internal organization of this hospital. Between 1950 and 1958 Dr. Harold Wise pioneered the idea of a health care team to provide more personalized and less fragmented care.[20] The team "would consist of a series of professionals trained to manage the interpersonal aspects of social situations, and to use data from a variety of sources and transmit it appropriately,"[21] or in the words of a general medical text, physicians would become team leaders and "concentrate on the more difficult aspects [of health care] such as identifying problems from the data base and organizing approaches to these problems, while assigning more routine tasks to other members of the team."[22] Medicine would sit atop the hierarchy of sciences and provide a "means to promote information flow among the science disciplines by providing a common subject for investigation and a common language."[23] The physician's responsibility "would be not only to the individual patient, but to the variety of levels of society implicated in the disease processes,"[24] and medicine would expand over the length and breadth of human activity, collecting, analyzing and routing information as any good management team should.

The hospital penetrates into the community through screening programs designed to find those people who might have an illness but who do not experience themselves as "sick." "[Multiple screening] means the application of a battery of economical, rapidly applied tests to screen out apparently well persons who probably have a disease from those who probably do not. The fact that many chronic diseases develop insidiously to the danger point, the fact that the same individual may have several chronic diseases detectable by laboratory tests, the fact that these tests are most economical when applied on a sizable scale—these facts support the extension of multiple screening, not only in physician's offices but also in hospitals and health centers."[25] Perhaps the most interesting recent extension of medicine outside of the hospital involves screening for hypertension. Supported by a massive television ad campaign, people who have hypertension are urged to take their medicine by the slogan "do it for the loved ones in your life" while others are encouraged to monitor their own blood pressure using machines located in shopping centers and banks. This kind of screening program does not even require trained personnel, just technology and vigorous marketing.

The principal aim of current discussions is integration of services so that patients do not interfere with the new medical practice as they did with the old medical practice in hospitals. The Commission on Chronic Illness took as one its goals "to suggest patterns for desirable relationships between services, facilities, and programs." "Good integration and coordination of services and facilities is one of the most promising means of assuring" that the social aspects of care are met, the Commission said.[26] Medical and community services need to be integrated. "There should be close administrative, professional, and geographical ties between a general hospital and all other facilities and services for the chronically ill, including home care services. Services should be organized so that patients can move easily to and from home, hospital, and nursing home."[27] Ease and smooth functioning become the indicators of quality in medical care systems.

Internally, the practice of medicine changed as well. Since the late 1960s texts have encouraged physicians to write problem-oriented medical records instead of records oriented toward diagnosis and treatment of specific, identifiable diseases. *Harrison's Principles of Internal Medicine* says, "the patient's record must be designed so that it expresses specifically what physicians deal with most frequently—the *problems* of patients." This text is gently critical of the old disease-oriented method of inquiry. "While the ultimate goal of clinical taxonomy is directed toward identification of etiology, pathology, and pathologic physiology, in view of their importance as guides to therapy, it would be both unrealistic and dangerous to require a specific diagnosis for severely dyspneic patients [people who subjectively experience difficulty in breathing] in the absence of reasonably convincing information concerning the reason for dyspnea. Until the cause can be established, all diagnostic modalities and therapeutic interventions are oriented to the real and immediate problem—dyspnea."[28] Dyspnea, in the old taxonomic approach to medical inquiry, was a symptom. It was often thought to have a strong psychological component and thus was often brushed aside as psychosomatic or "unreal." But dyspnea is a disruption in the structure of the holon. It limits one's range of movement and restricts one's exercise. The person experiencing shortness of breath, with or without an organic "cause," no longer fits into the pattern of things as he or she did before. Dyspnea may remain, in one sense, a symptom of more fundamental problems, but under the new medical logic it is accorded co-equal status with the heart disease that may underlie it. Regardless of its underlying cause, dyspnea is a problem. Within the purview of the new medical logic it has become real in and of itself, commands attention, and compels action.

Even the more traditional "Johns Hopkins" text, *The Principles and Practice of Modern Medicine,* a book that traces its heritage to Sir William Osler's nineteenth century medical text, tells the physician to worry more about locating a person who has problems in terms of his or her history and life circumstances—in terms of relationships—than about naming the disease causing the problem. "It is as important to understand the person afflicted by the disease as it is to understand the disease afflicting the person. Information about both [is] obtained at the same time. The patient's attitude, demeanor, and appearance all give the perceptive physician insights into the patient as does the way in which the patient relates to the physician."[29] The text plays down the importance of the differential diagnosis, an iterative binary choice procedure that uses specific tests or procedures to collect data that allow one to discard some possible diagnoses of a patient's condition and retain others until only one diagnosis remains. In place of this classical approach to medical inquiry the text recommends "the rapid iteration of the diagnostic process throughout the encounter with the patient,"[30] an almost intuitive process of hypothesis formation, search for data in the patient's life, and reformation of one's hypothesis or tentative diagnosis. This process forces the physician to search for information, facts in context, data which have meaning as a result of their relations to other data.

By "humanizing" the patient-physician encounter, by becoming concerned and interested, by being sensitive, unbiased and non-judgmental, the experienced physician can come to know a patient's life, locate facts derived from the history, physical examination, and laboratory tests in the dynamic space in which the patient lives, and thereby convert data into information. In turn, "information may prompt the physician to take certain actions, actions which may include seeking further information," but which must be directed toward "the whole purpose of clinical information analysis—the solution of a patient's problem."[31] The patient with a problem, defined in terms of the patient's entire life, has displaced the disease—a visible thing displayed before the physician's informed gaze—as the object of medical attention.

The traditional physician worked on diseases. If the notion of disease has changed and been replaced by patient's problems, the question naturally arises, "What does the new physician do?" How do doctors respond to problems once diseases have lost their privileged position in medical thought?

The modern physician manages patients who bring their problems to him. Treating disease is subsumed under management. "Patient management involves far more than treatment. Indeed, it involves more than managing the patient's illness. *Treatment* implies the application of one or several therapeutic measures. *Management* is directed toward designing and implementing the most effective program of care for the particular patient's total problem."[32] The physician must take the total situation of the patient into consideration in order to put the patient's life course on a normal if not optimal trajectory. Harrison's text says, "it is the duty of the physician to guide the patient through an illness."[33]

A systems-theoretic approach to medical care encourages the physician to look to more complex levels of the holon hierarchy of systems for the perturbations that are now identified with "disease" and for approaches to patient management different from those suggested by a strictly organic/organismic theory of disease. "Management . . . takes cognizance of personal and social factors, such as the role of the patient's chronic alcoholism or the impact of hospitalization on his employment. Furthermore, management includes recognition of a home situation which may preclude effective implementation of a therapeutic plan outside the hospital."[34] In fact, systems theory conceives of management schemes as perturbations in the holon hierarchy and suggests these schemes are conceptually equivalent to diseases. The difference between a disease and therapy is that therapeutic management schemes are supposed to restore the original patterns of the array of systems which were disrupted by the original perturbation, the disease. "Intrinsically, therapies and the causes of disease are both perturbations. . . . The difference between disease perturbations and therapies lies in the value judgment placed on the presumed outcome of their impact upon the hierarchy."[35] So the modern physician interferes in a patient's life in order to restore order after the patient identifies a disorder as problematic. And the physician interferes in an ongoing fashion to insure the patient's life follows an unproblematic course.

The problem-oriented medical record governs patient management. It contains, first of all, a data base taken from the medical history, the physical examination, and laboratory tests. The data base is the background against which any problem or any datum acquires meaning. It is the basis for locating the patient. Second, the record contains a problem list. "It should contain those features in the patient's psychobiological makeup that require continuing attention by the physician and other members of the health team. Thus the list must contain entries relating to social history (e.g., marital discord), risk factors (e.g., familial polyposis of the colon), symptoms. . . , physical findings. . . , laboratory tests. . . , etc."[36]

Just as the museum curator tries to convey the richness of an ecology in the museum tableaux without displaying all the elements of an ecology, the physician must be selective in constructing a problem list. One must approach the problem list as one approaches the limited space of the tableau, with "a sense of proportion, so that a variety of minor, self-limited problems (e.g., colds, sprains, minor gastrointestinal upsets) are excluded from the master problem list, which might otherwise be unduly cluttered with trivial illnesses."[37] The well written record details the logic of one's approach to each problem. It includes the patient's interpretation of his or her problem, associated data, the physician's interpretation of the meaning of the data, and a management plan. Then the record follows the patient's course toward resolution of problems, toward living with them, or to the patient's death. Data flow sheets sequentially follow problems ammenable to quantification and regular assessment. The master problem list serves as an index to the rest of the record in which progress notes indicate the course of a problem that cannot be followed with simple, regular tests.

Problem-oriented records, however, are more than simply records of data interpretations, plans, and outcomes. Records actually structure and control medical work. They force physicians to think well and they organize allied health personnel to insure that every potential approach to a patient's problem is considered. "The requirement that all members of the health team systematically display their thoughts and actions improves communication and potentiates supervision. . . . Furthermore, the establishment of a plan for each problem leads to clearer assignment of specific tasks to each of [the health team's] members."[38] Patient management involves all of the relationships shown in Figure 6.1, and the prob-

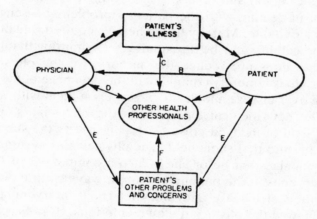

FIGURE 6.1 The multiple interactions that occur between the various people (ellipses) and problems (rectangles). There is a tendency to focus on the interactions shown by the bold arrows. Good management requires attention to all of the interactions. Reproduced, with permission, from A. McGehee Harvey et al., eds., *The Principles and Practice of Modern Medicine*, 20th ed., New York: Appleton-Century-Crofts, 1980, p. 12.

lem-oriented record insures that all the relationships in the figure receive attention, not just the relationship between the doctor and the patient's illness (line A), which formed the basis of traditional medical work.

The systems–theoretic–ecological–problem–oriented approach to medicine reorganizes medical care. One theoretical article went so far as to say that under the new approach "the physician would . . . cease to exist as such." Under the new medical logic, "the physician would be a systems manager"[39] who, like a factory manager, would insure that data are collected and pertinent parts of a person's life are monitored, and who would send out information (via the medical record) that certain adjustments in the patient's holon hierarchy of systems need to be made.

The new logic causes the physician to become a person. The physician as person is subject to all the human problems faced by the patient-person and others. "The young physician may feel inadequate in dealing with the patient's problems; a sense of insecurity is inevitable. Moreover, the newly acquired role of authority and responsibility may be threatening."[40] Admitting that physicians are people does not reduce the authority of the physician; nor, however, does it merely complement the old image of the physician hovering over disease and death, gazing upon them with well trained eyes. The new medical logic inserts the physician's subjectivity into the field of medical power just as it inserts the subjectivity of the patient into that same field. The physician as systems manager must recognize that he or she is also a component of the system that intervenes in the patient's holon in ways counteractive to the intervention of disease and that the whole intervening system— including now the physician's own emotions, desires, personality, character, class, and culture—must be monitored and controlled. The technical skills of the physician, controlled through training in medical school and practice in the clinic, are to be complemented with interpersonal skills controlled through "humaneness, a sense of confidence and security based upon the conviction that all will be done that can be done."[41]

In the expansion of the object of medical interest from the disease to the holon and the concomitant change of the role of the physician and the organization of medical care, what has happened to the patient? The patient expanded into a person around 1950, as the body lost its privileged place in medical thinking, but medicine has recreated the person as a hierarchy of systems within a larger hierarchy of systems. Has the person now lost the privileged place granted it when it replaced the patient? Is the person simply to lapse back into what he had been for nearly two hundred years, namely, no more than a locus for disease? The answer is no. In fact, quite the opposite has happened. The person has been elevated in medical thinking to the status of health team member, joint adventurer, co-worker.

From a systems-theoretical point of view the individual is important because "the Person, like the atom, represents a naturally stable point in the hierarchy. . . . Death of the individual sets off a domino-like destruction of all subcomponent levels down to the atoms and simple molecules, while the individual can often survive the breakups of family, community, or nation."[42] But the individual is important for other reasons as well. The meaning the person gives to his or her situation is the point of departure in the new medical encounter. The patient's problems initiate medical inquiry. Problems are central and become the basis of the medical record, but the physician is urged to place the patient well above the record: "A possible danger of the [problem-oriented medical record] is that the emotional needs of patients may receive even less attention from a busy physician who is intent on writing excellent notes. The patient and not the record must remain the primary focus of physician care."[43] Some people follow the emergent importance of the individual down a path that takes them perilously close to destruction of the traditional structure of the medical encounter. Thus, for example, Howard Brody said that one of the implications for medicine of a systems perspective is that "a model of medical practice for the future must have as a central feature the shifting of decision making back to the patient, as much as possible."[44] In a similar vein Ivan Illich wants to "de-institutionalize" medicine along with the rest of society.[45] Instead of following its new logic in this direction, though, medicine has tried to restructure the doctor-patient relationship.

One group of pediatricians based their proposals for a new relationship on the recognition that the holon hierarchy of systems exists in an environment of limited resources. They argue that options are constrained, and unrestricted individual choice cannot be permitted. "The health and health care prerogatives of any individual," they say, "must be constrained by the sharing of responsibility for them with the rest of society. Individual pursuit of one's own best interests may bring ruin to us all."[46] They and others[47] have embraced Garrett Hardin's notion that we all share a "commons,"[48] a limited set of resources available to the community that must be protected from the ravages of individual choice by collective decisions to control access to the commons. If health care is a "commons," it can be protected only if patients and physicians accept joint responsibility for making health care decisions with ultimate respect not for the individual, not for the patient, and not for health, but for the commons. Shared responsibility must, according to this view, be organized so that the continued existence of the holon is insured and its orderly set of internal relationships is minimally disrupted.

Different texts describe the mission of medicine differently, but the varied descriptions tend to converge on one theme: physician and patient join together in a search for an optimal life strategy which respects a distant, somewhat vague idea of the social order that is part of the normative structure of life. Physicians "want to move the patients [they] serve toward, or maintain them at, some mutually agreed and acceptable levels of behavior and function."[49] So physicians negotiate the nature of care with patients, alleviate "all conditions that 'limit life in its powers, enjoyment, and duration,' "[50] but maintain "active concern [for] the social, political, and economic processes which affect the health care system within which the patient seeks care and cure."[51] With the rise of the individual, medicine's field of power expands. The mission of medicine remains the same, but the scope of medicine's interests enlarges and presents medicine with new challenges. "Seen in this light, the care of the social body as a whole presents new and exciting challenges to the medical profession; it constitutes an enlargement of its calling."[52]

The expression of power within this enlarged calling is a double-edged sword. On the one hand, in ways different from those of traditional medicine, medical power controls patients. On the other hand, medical power controls medicine. Under the new practices of medical discourse the patient gains a voice and is no longer strictly "spoken for" by the physician. Yet the patient's voice is not a voice that speaks strictly for itself either. Both the patient and the physician must speak in concert toward a common end, a joint adventure.

Talcott Parsons wrote in general terms in 1969 about the special nature of the modern professional-client relationship. It is not, he pointed out, a market relationship governed by the principle of *caveat emptor*. Instead, it is organized around three social functions: the utilization of knowledge toward some practical end (curing the patient, for example); the creation of new knowledge (research); and, sometimes, the transmission of knowledge (teaching). The patient does not pay the physician for health, per se; the patient pays an entry fee for admission to the relationship through which all three of these social functions are pursued. In such a situation opportunities for exploitation and other manifestations of professional power arise. To avoid this, Parsons argued in his indirectly normative way, "a 'professional' element must establish an appropriate pattern of relationship to a 'lay' element. . . . [Clients] must, by and large, be brought into some kind of membership status with the professional personnel, in common solidary collective structures."[53] In short, patients must be made members of the health care team.

This sounds good, but a health care team that has patients as members requires a rather sophisticated system of control over all of its members. Difficult as that may sound, it is a problem medicine has addressed.

Under medicine's new logic, the patient-physician relationship is constructed so that the patient can and will speak the truth about his or her problems. The patient must conceal nothing, and it is the task of medicine to see that the patient can fulfill his or her obligations in the encounter. The "Johns Hopkins" text offers these recommendations for helping the patient provide essential information:

1. Make the patient comfortable, both physically and mentally. . . .

2. Make certain that the patient knows who you are and understands your role in his care. . . .

3. In general, interview the patient alone. . . .

4. Give the patient the conviction that he has a warm and understanding listener and adequate time in which to tell his whole story. . . .

5. . . . At the outset, afford the patient enough time to express in his own terms, without interruption, his basic reason for visiting you. . . .

8. Encourage the patient to use his own words, and not simply to recite diagnoses and interpretations of other physicians.

9. Never make the patient feel inadequate, dull, or distraught. If a particular line of questioning makes the patient embarrassed or anxious, move on to another topic without pressing too far at the time of the initial encounter. However, it is wise to explore that topic later once rapport has been established, for such behavior may indicate significant information lies in that area. . . .

12. The patient must be requestioned as the illness proceeds and new information evolves. . . .[54]

The details of a patient's life must be revealed by the patient so that the physician can use that information to insure that the management scheme devised for the patient optimizes his or her life course. The patient side of the patient-physician dyad is disciplined, but it is a discipline that involves a participant in a joint adventure and can no longer place the patient under a rule of silence.

We need to recognize, however, that disciplining the patient is effected only by disciplining the physician. After all, the instructions outlined above are instructions *to the physician* and concern the physician's demeanor. Under the new regime, medicine does not stand outside of the medical gaze. The field of medical power is reflexive. It encompasses not only the patient (or the extended holon) but medicine itself.

Examples of the reflexivity of the medical gaze abound after 1970. Compliance researchers, for example, quickly learned that it might not be the health beliefs of patients that determine compliance with prescribed regimens of care; but, on the contrary, it might be compliance with prescribed regimens of care that determines health beliefs.[55] This turned medical inquiry around. Instead of asking what about the patient made the patient compliant, medicine had to look at itself and ask what about medicine made the patient compliant? Medicine became introspective. "In the last analysis, the physician-patient relationship may well be the most crucial variable in determining compliance with treatment plans. In the daily work of the busy practitioner, failure to take the time for truly adequate communication is probably the most common and damaging deficiency of modern medicine."[56] This understanding of failure does not locate the problem in a defective or unruly personality of the patient. It blames the manager for not structuring relationships properly and for not insuring that information flows properly through the system.

As another example, consider contemporary concerns about malpractice. Texts tell physicians that in order to avoid malpractice suits and provide good care, all that is necessary is "good management." The physician who attends to the relationship, communicates well, helps the patient communicate deep-seated concerns, fears, anxieties, and desires, who is introspective and critical of his or her own ability, and who records everything accurately need not fear a charge of negligence.[57] The systems logic that now informs medicine pivots on the old logic and charges medicine to be introspective to such a degree that one text said, "Above all, perhaps, we must understand ourselves well so that we do not assume any degree of privilege and responsibility that is rightly the patient's."[58]

If physicians will not be thoughtfully introspective and discipline themselves, their professional milieu will do it for them. There are means for disciplining physicians other than the ritualistic ceremonies of confession before one's peers discussed by Bosk.[59] The problem-oriented medical record, we are told, "reveals the process of patient care in a manner that can be evaluated." It "set[s] the stage for a lifelong educational process of self and peer evaluation through effective record audit."[60]

Even medicine's technology cuts both ways today. For example, a new procedure called thermography can detect painful areas of the body. Thermographs are pictures of the body that show small variations in the surface temperature of the body. In them painful areas appear several degrees cooler than normal. A *New York Times* article on the procedure acclaimed it by saying, "Pain victims who have been told by doctors that the suffering is 'all in your head' may have a new ally in thermography." The pain victim presumably can use thermographic data to legitimate his or her complaint to a physician who, for whatever reason, is not able to find a "real reason" for the pain. Only late in the *New York Times* article are we told "the method is expected not only to aid true sufferers but to weed out malingerers who are getting undeserved disability pay."[61] We might read this cynically and think that the "patient's ally" argument is just a public relations ploy designed to gain wider acceptance for a technique whose "real" purpose is to save the capitalist state a bit of money by detecting those who might leech off it, but this would be unfair. New medical technologies together with the new doctor-patient relationship characterized by dialogue and negotiation allow patients to monitor doctors' actions just as doctors monitor patients' statuses. If the patient and medicine are to be participants in a joint adventure that conforms to the normative structures of life as they are understood by medicine, then patient and physician must speak at least in overlapping languages if not in a common language. If the patient must make visible his or her deepest self in terms of a language comprehensible to medicine, the physician must bring his or her technology out of the shadows of mystery and share it with the patient. Ever finer assessment devices whose data are used to illuminate patients' problems rather that to diagnose esoteric diseases can be read and understood by patients or patient advocates and can be used to control physicians just as physicians use the same data to control patients.

How are we to understand this new medical revolution? We believe we are witnessing a great reversal in medicine. Once, as Ariès has shown, considerable work was devoted to the task of taming death. Death was the great beast that stalked in the darkness and that threatened to attack unannounced at any moment. Now, in a Frankensteinian reversal, the great beast is no longer death but life. Life and living threaten, not death and dying. It is the lives of patients that present the most difficult medical issues today; their deaths are just special management problems.

# Seven

# The Joint Adventure:
# Birthing, Aging, Dying

Sometime in the fifteenth or sixteenth century, the *Oxford English Dictionary* says, the word *adventure* "passed insensibly" from meaning a chance event, something that happens without design, or "a hazardous or perilous enterprise or performance" into meaning "any novel or unexpected event in which one shares." Jean-Paul Sartre showed us how the term has been pushed through the remainder of a 180-degree change of meaning in the twentieth century when he had Antoine Roquentin talk about adventures and his life in *Nausea*. "I haven't had any adventures," Roquentin says. "Things have happened to me, events, incidents, anything you like. But not adventures." Roquentin is not exactly sure what an adventure would be or what he wants that would constitute an adventure but he says, "anyway, I had imagined that at certain moments my life could take on a rare and precious quality. There was no need for extraordinary circumstances: all I asked for was a little order."[1] Much later, he reflects on how people in his world recognize an adventure if they are sharing in one: "all of a sudden you feel that time is passing, that each moment leads to another moment, this one to yet another and so on. . . ."[2] Modern adventures are written backwards, the last event being known or expected and pointing back to inform all that precedes it; an event becomes part of an adventure only when it anticipates and points directly to the next event, and the next, and the next, to the very end event, the close of the adventure. An adventure, Roquentin says, "achieves significance only through its death."[3] Instead of being a matter of happenstance, the modern adventure is a reconstructed series of events, the first of which points to the last and the last of which imparts meaning to the first.

Carried by its new logic modern medicine proposes to become the author of the modern adventure of life. Modern medicine arose in opposition to death and offered patients the possibility of life. After 1950, under its "expanded calling," medicine began to build the basis for offering patients not just the possibility of life, but life itself. Medicine became the mediator of the true life, the fulfilled life, the managerially optimized life. As medicine's attention shifted away from disease and toward the person, its goal shifted away from health and toward life. It began to map life which came to be identified with the trajectories people follow from conception to death, and to develop a calculus of optimal trajectories together with analyses of deviations from those trajectories. Birth as a momentous and revelatory event and birth as a play of force and counterforce in the body tend to vanish and give way to "birthing," the process. Death as a momentous and revelatory event similarly gives way to "dying," the process. Each have been studied in painful detail and one is connected to the other by the equally carefully analyzed "life cycle." Together these processes form the skeletal structure of an adventure in which the newborn's first breath, carefully monitored and managed, anticipates its last just as the first sentence of a finely constructed adventure story anticipates the final scene.

Medicine does not practice its knowledge of life's processes in the same way it used its knowledge of life's events. Knowledge of birth, something that happened to women, led to the controlling brutality of obstetrical forceps and prophylactic episiotomies so that the event of birth, when it happened, did not cause anything else to happen. Knowledge of birthing, something women experience and in which they participate, is not used to control women in the old fashion way. Instead, birthing is held up as an ideal, a vision of the desirable but typically unreachable. People may choose to try to approximate the ideal, and, if they so choose, medicine will help them achieve an optimal birthing trajectory.

It is not a question of medicine forcing an individual to choose an optimal path; for, alongside the map of the ideal life course, medicine has developed the parallel line of thought that mandates respect for the individual. Medicine does not bludgeon people to conform to the optimal life course. It merely sits between these parallel tracks—the map of the good life from birth to death and the course chosen by the willful, free, inviolable individual—and offers the latter assistance in achieving the former. Medicine offers the individual a share in the adventure it has written. It offers people the opportunity to become joint adventurers.

An intense commitment to mapping the minute details of life arose only recently. Nineteenth century obstetrics, for example, thought of birth as a delimited event which consisted of three distinct stages. During the first stage, contractions gradually built up as the cervix softened and dilated somewhat. Then women experienced a transition to the second stage, a lull in contractions followed by forceful labor of a different character from that during the first stage. The second stage ended with the expulsion of the fetus and the third, or placental, stage began. After the expulsion of the placenta, birth—the event—was over. In the 1950s the stages of birth gave way to a calculus of birth. Emmanuel Friedman mapped the instant-to-instant changes in cervical dilatation over time and plotted an "ideal" labor progress curve, a mean labor progress curve, and statistical deviations around those curves. Many obstetrical difficulties could be understood in terms of Friedman's "partographs." Friedman traced the implications of different partographic trajectories and also developed technology to monitor cervical dilatation over time.[4]

Friedman's work contained both the individualizing map of each woman's own, unique progress through labor and the map of an ideal course with which, presumably, the woman in labor could be aligned by the use of various technologies. Other aspects of birth were reconceptualized to stress their continuous character and new technologies sprung up around the new ideas. The fetal monitor, a machine that measures uterine contractions and fetal heart rate simultaneously and continuously, is but a small part of the obstetrician's array of devices for monitoring and optimizing the birth process.[5] In general, the transformation of medical discourse that occurred in 1950 required that new concepts and technologies embody the parallel lines of medical thought, the carefully monitored individual and the ideal course determined through study of the maps of many individual courses.

More recently dying has been mapped. Elisabeth Kübler-Ross's *On Death and Dying* is the acknowledged ground-breaking work in this effort.[6] She suggested that the terminally ill pass through several stages once they learn they are dying. First, they are shocked and deny that they could be dying. Then they become angry, perhaps try to bargain their way out of their situation, and then they become depressed when they realize the impossibility of success. Finally, they grieve for their anticipated loss of their own life, and then, if they get to the final stage, they accept death peacefully. Kübler-Ross's stages of dying incited considerable research which showed, variously, that many people do pass through these stages or that people jump through the stages in odd orders, or that the stages sometimes overlap one another. In a parallel development Glaser and Strauss suggested that the "trajectory" of the dying person's life might be a useful conceptual tool for understanding and studying the terminally ill.[7]

The desire to construct a map of dying persisted and was extended. In 1975 Raymond Moody published his controversial *Life After Life*, which suggested that people who survive a near-death experience pass through a common set of experiences or stages that involves separation from the body, passage through a tunnel or other conveyance to another world, participation in a "light" that characterizes the other world, and finally, after a review of one's life on earth, the decision to return to this world.[8] To Moody and people who have done similar work, the individual experiences of near-death survivors suggest a common course for the dying who pass Kübler-Ross's stages. Furthermore, they suggest an ideal course for those who can manage to die well. For example, researchers tell us people who attempt suicide do not have the pleasurable near-death experiences of people who almost die by "natural causes."

Medicine has accepted the stages-of-dying theory and urges its incorporation into the care of the dying, the patients the "Johns Hopkins" text terms "a special management problem." Physician's texts tell them to be aware of the stages because "insight into these stages permits the physician to deal with the real issues better."[9] The anger shown the technician who causes great pain when taking blood or the anger shown the orderly who pushes the wheelchair too fast is not *real* anger with the technician or with the orderly, the texts suggest; it is anger directed at the patient's own situation. Stages-of-dying theories give a physician a purchase on the "real," admitting the subjectivity of the person into medical discourse but in such a way that it meshes well with the medically determined structure of that discourse.

It is not clear yet what medicine will do with stage theories of near-death experiences; but Kenneth Ring, a psychologist who studied over one hundred people brought back from the brink of death, believes that accounts of near death experiences can reduce anxiety in other people about to die, can be used to prevent suicide (since suicide attempters have different and less rich experiences) and can be used as the basis for establishing a "Center for the Dying Person," a facility that would be better than a hospice.[10]

Death is offered as the apotheosis of life. We are back, in a way, to the theme lost less than 200 years ago. Life gains meaning through death, but only in a way. Dying, like birthing, has become a phenomenon that exists between the individual and the ideal, between the experiential and the socially optimal. "The dying process is deeply personal, yet it is also a social phenomenon. It is totally individualistic, yet it is shared, and generalizations can be made about it," we are told.[11] Dying becomes, thus, part of the adventure of life mapped by medicine. Certainly, research on dying is being used as the backward pointer every adventure needs at its end. Kenneth Ring, for example, says, "To live in the shadow of death, as if each day may be our last, can clearly promote a quickening of one's spiritual sensitivity. Pettiness and selfishness recede; expressions of love and compassion are natural to this state."[12] And Richard Kalish wants to turn the old saw "We begin to die the moment we begin to live" around to say "We begin to live the moment we begin to die."[13]

If we can be permitted to propose our own set of stages, we would say that medicine has passed through three stages in the construction of death. First, death was "my death," to use Ariès's phrase. Each individual stood in intimate relation with his or her own death, which was invisible to others. Then medicine made death visible and entered the era of "death produced" by hostile, invading substances and forces that left traces in the body visible only to the physician. Now dying has become a doubly privileged last stage of life. It is doubly privileged because it tells us how well we have managed our lives, and it tells us about what we can do to tie up some of the loose ends of lives that have not been optimally managed. Now we live in an era of the "regulated and well managed death" that is the final stage of life. We do not purport to tame death today; instead, we manage dying in order to tame life.

Aging connects birthing and dying. Concept development, data collection, and theory formulation on the "life cycle" have occurred primarily outside of medicine, but the "life cycle" concept has become an organizing feature of many medical school curricula. Texts alert physicians to developmental problems typically associated with one stage of life or another. Medicine has long appreciated the problems of infancy, childhood, and adolescence, but the life cycle perspective extends the physician's interest to problems associated with work, early adult life (the period when one explores intimate relationships and perhaps decides to have children), midlife (the period when childrearing pressures lessen and retirement approaches), and the period after retirement.[14] A life course perspective integrates the work of disciplines peripheral to medicine whose contributions are nonetheless essential if medicine is to meet the demands of its expanded calling.

During the 1970s the life cycle perspective formed around several simple propositions about aging: (1) one ages from birth (or conception) to death; (2) aging is biological, psychological, and sociological, and the three dimensions of aging must be understood interactively, not separately; (3) social forces affect life courses of individuals and of cohorts of people born during a specified period who age together; and (4) the way people or cohorts of people age affects society and often effects social change.[15] There is nothing profound in this perspective. The propositions on which it is based are simply a restatement of the systems-theoretic view of the person as an interactive, hierarchically integrated, dynamic set of systems. The perspective is crucial to medicine, though, because "aging" and the "life cycle" become the conceptual infrastructure for constructing maps of life. With birthing, aging, and dying, medicine obtains an integrated conceptual hold on living.

Medicine's maps are arrayed alongside the other pole of the new medical logic, which emphasizes the individual and elevates subjective experience to the realm of the medically real. These two very different lines of thought have developed simultaneously. They are not contradictory as they might seem at first glance. They form an ambiguity around which medical practice is being refashioned. Medicine is no longer that distant, professionally closeted expert that sallies forth to meet disease and death wherever they show themselves. Medicine is now one of the omni-present, unaggressive modern experts of whom Jacques Donzelot wrote, "You find them because you look for them, but they do not come looking for you; they do not come to your home as a social worker or educator would do. . . . They hold out the possibility of achieving, through their help, a freedom from constraints, from the heaviness of customs, from the arbitrariness of rules. . . . They will help you rediscover the true path your life should follow, for a few bills and a dash of those images that prowl about in our psyches."[16] The new medical logic organizes medical power around the practices of monitoring. Medicine monitors individual lives, extracts individuality—those images prowling about inside, sorts through that individuality for indications of deviations from carefully mapped optimal life courses, locates individuals precisely in terms of those deviations, and then offers freedom from those deviations in the form of a true and fulfilling life course. Medicine frees individuals from the problems of their individuality through techniques of normalization.

The "chronic patient," again, is the symbol of this new perspective. The new logic, first, makes constantly visible that which was previously invisible to medicine: "the handicapped was truly the forgotten and neglected man. The condition of these unfortunate individuals was deplored, but little or nothing was done about them except for an insufficient amount of charity."[17] Second, this logic makes the "whole" person an object of medical attention even when asymptomatic and exposes the "whole" person to "comprehensive" health management schemes: "Practitioners, institutions, and programs . . . have an obligation to apply early diagnosis and prompt and comprehensive treatment of the whole patient to prevent or postpone deteriorations and complications. . . ."[18] Third, it individualizes the whole person. The person is no longer a member of a class of sick people or even of a class of people with a specific disease. "Of great importance in its implications for future action was the oft-repeated tenet that the long-term patient needs to be looked on as an individual, whole person." "Coordination [of services] helps greatly . . . in preventing fractionation of the patient by different specialist interests."[19] Medicine individualizes by identifying people as unique collections of "deviations from normal."[20] Fourth, this apparatus emphasizes the notion of rehabilitation, which seeks to reintegrate the individual into technically useful places in society. As this idea was summarized by the President's Commission on Chronic Illness in 1957, "Rehabilitation is 'the restoration of the handicapped to the fullest physical, mental, social, vocational and economic usefulness of which they are capable.' It requires total evaluation of the individual from many standpoints and undertaking a program of treatment aimed at maximum recovery. If it is to be fully effective, the idea of 'total care' should pervade all treatment efforts, from the time the patient first consults a physician until every possible thing has been accomplished.''[21]

In his introduction to Georges Canguilhem's *On the Normal and the Pathological,* Michel Foucault wrote, "At life's most basic level, the play of code and decoding leaves room for chance, which before being disease, deficit or monstrosity, is something like perturbation in the information system, something like a 'mistake.' In the extreme, life is that which is capable of error."[22] The power of nineteenth century medicine created out of error the anomaly and opposed it to the normal while the parallel power whose face was compassion took the anomaly out of the dark fringes of society and integrated the opposition into the social. The anomaly, to be sure, was carefully isolated within the social—it was an outcast on the inside—but compassion gave the anomaly a place, its true place. The power of contemporary medicine creates the individual out of error. Mid-century medicine created the individual who was not just *an example* of life, which, in general, is "capable of error," but was an intimately known, highly individuated collection of errors that is opposed to nothing.

For those who live under the power of contemporary medicine this means, in figurative terms, we are all Elephant Men like John Merrick. The concept of "chronic disease" and the practice that surrounds it extend to everyone the power of the new medical gaze. The 1957 report of the Commission on Chronic Illness began, "Chronic disease is a problem whose scope is as great as the total population of the country."[23] This statement echoed the sentiments expressed by Ernst Boas seventeen years earlier: "There is hardly a family, one member of which is not stricken by some illness such as heart disease, rheumatism, cancer or diabetes."[24] On both "humanitarian [and] economic grounds"[25] everyone is now subject to medical and social control—both cure and care, assessment, amelioration of symptoms *and* proper placement—of an expanded medical discourse on life. In the name of tolerance and acceptance, medicine makes the anomalous and the different into people who are socially useful. Speaking of a book on chronic illness in children, R. J. Haggerty said: "This book will help us move toward the day when we can assist all children to reach their full potential, when we and society can accept the handicapped, value their strengths, and not demand all children be alike and perfect, else we relegate them to places out-of-sight, out-of-mind. This is perhaps the greatest lesson to be learned from this book—tolerance of differences and addition of skills to the physician who wishes to help those who are different to lead more effective lives."[26] The task of modern medicine, it seems, is to titrate its own deployment so that medical power is totalizing, integrative, and rapidly responsive to every nuance on the social horizon while, at the same time, it remains unobtrusive, "humane," even "liberating."

The social form that achieves this and that is the starting point for the joint adventure in medicine is the support group. The support group synthesizes all aspects of the techniques of normalization. It provides a judgmentally benign arena in which individuality can be aired. Indeed, it is a social form that demands expression of individuality, all those minor, intimate, hidden details of life that facilitate or stand in the way of the good life. Second, the support group contains knowledge of the trajectories that constitute the good life. Third, the support group provides a forum in which the expert and the individual can join together in order to make the concerns and anxieties of the patient inert by invoking positive imagery and normalizing technologies. Many support groups are paramedical. They form at the periphery of the clinic and are run by "lay experts" who have special knowledge, training, or experience in a particular aspect of personal development. However, the support group is the model for the new medical encounter. It is the form that ties together the two lines of modern medical thought—that which individualizes and that which maps—and the form that joins together the individual, with his or her unique, special concerns and problems, and the expert whose knowledge is redemptive.

Support groups for birthing are familiar. Natural childbirth is the term we generally associate with several different approaches to obstetrical care that have in common their respect for the psychological aspects of childbirth. The psychoprophylactic school that traces its origins to the hypnotic approach to birth developed in Russia in the early part of the century and follows its heritage across Europe to the practice of Lamaze in France stresses techniques of psychological conditioning to relieve childbirth pain and anxiety. Yet these psychological techniques are learned, practiced, and employed in support groups. Women are taught exercises, and psychologically and physiologically beneficial breathing techniques, and are conditioned to anticipate, understand, and control their bodies' functions throughout birth. Then, in labor, women use the techniques under the watchful eye of a *monitrice,* labor coach, or supportive companion who has been trained to note deviations from the prescribed regimen and signs of distress or tiring and to insure that each woman keeps her own vigil over her own behavior.

The other major school of natural childbirth traces its roots to the work of Grantly Dick-Read.[27] Dick-Read felt that advanced cultures educated women to fear childbirth and that fear led to tension which, in turn, led to pain. Dick-Read proposed educational efforts to counter the influence of culture and society. His romantic, even spiritual, images of pregnancy and birth permeated the antenatal literature of the post–World War II period[28] and various organizations formed support groups to tell women that birth could be beautiful if only they would vocalize, recognize, and then counter their innermost hesitations about reproduction.

The romanticism of Dick-Read led in an unbroken line to the psychosexual approach to childbirth promulgated by Sheila Kitzinger.[29] Her approach recognizes that "women express their own personalities with infinite variety in childbirth,"[30] but simultaneously Kitzinger's method holds out the promise of the ultimate birth experience. Through proper education and by cultivating proper relationships with counselors, attendants, and supporters, the delivering woman can learn to trust her body, surrender to it completely as she does in lovemaking, and achieve a wonderful and even orgasmic birth.[31]

Obstetrics recognized almost immediately the value—the obstetrical value—of natural childbirth, particularly those aspects of it that go under the heading of "support." Dr. Herbert Thoms said in 1951, for example, " 'support' during active labor is the most important single factor in our [preparation for childbirth] program."[32] Support meant then, as it does now, making sure that a woman is subjected to a constant field of visibility. "As nearly as possible, we try to have someone with the patient during her entire labor, whether it be a friend, nurse, husband, or intern."[33]

Visibility effects control and, if the field of visibility ever breaks down and a woman begins to lose control, there is no need to resort immediately to old regimens of control. Control can be reimplemented by fortifying the supportive field in which the woman is seen and knows she is on display and being judged against those optimal birthing trajectories she learned about during her pregnancy. One doctor praised the value of the visibility provided by "supportive settings" saying, "We have on many occasions been called to a patient who has lost control toward the end of labor. She was crying out with her contractions, thrashing about on the table in the intervals, thoroughly out of control. But after talking with her for a few minutes, sitting with her through a couple of contractions, reassuring her about the progress of her labor, we have been amazed to see this woman regain control, become relaxed and free of tension in the intervals, and bear down with her contractions with little evidence of the pain that had previously seemed so severe."[34]

The support group deploys a field of visibility which summons forth a discipline that aligns the individual with an obstetrically acceptable, if not ideal, labor course. And what a difference from the old means for effecting an obstetrically acceptable delivery!

The woman described above, out of control and thrashing about, was not brutalized; instead, she was reassured and joined in an adventure toward the wonderful climax of birthing which she knew was possible. Her experience of pain was normalized as her behavior was coaxed back onto an experientially optimizing, and yet managerially effective, birthing trajectory.

There are important parallels between the birthing literature and the dying literature. Lyn Lofland discusses what she calls the "Happy Death Movement" in her book, *The Craft of Dying: The Modern Face of Death*. Death's modern face is a benevolent, accepting, almost smiling face. At least that is the image proffered by the "sprawling, diverse, multi-structured, diffuse assemblage of persons . . . engaging in a multiplicity of largely uncoordinated activities" that form the movement.[35] The happy death movement suggests that dying and death can be periods of growth. They can be positive parts of life instead of being something into which one degenerates and which one experiences alone. Death can even be an orgasmic experience.[36] A modern orgasmic death is like a Masters and Johnson orgasm, the climax reached by following an externally inscribed, scientifically proper, carefully monitored, individually beneficial plan.

One achieves a happy death, according to the rhetoric of the movement, by expressing one's concerns. Just as natural childbirth classes "encourage women and their partners to *air their concerns* ahead of time"[37] so that their concerns can be met with trajectory adjusting technologies, the new approach to death tells the dying "that whatever the emotions engendered by dying and death, they *should be expressed*. To suppress expression is to sacrifice the opportunities for 'growth' which death provides. . . . Expressivity calls not simply for talk but for *talk about one's varying emotional states, which talk 'authentically' expresses those states*. Talk which is 'mere' intellectualizing is proscribed."[38] The real concerns of the individual must be published so that, with the help of others, the individual's dying course can be routed properly toward a good death.

The logic extends to survivors as well. Those left behind by the death of another are presumed to have a need to grieve. More than that, though, modern rhetoric suggests that grief has "an internally generated 'natural course' (it is a *process*) which, for the health of the actor, must be 'worked through.' "[39] With the help of experts and through the use of support group technologies the dying and those affected by another's death can achieve the good life right up to the moment of death.

To put such rhetoric into practice one simply needs to follow the implications of the logic discussed so far. First, the individual must be respected: "The terminally ill person's own framework of values, preferences and life-outlook must be taken into account in planning and conducting treatment. This is a standard which, in effect, maintains that treatment should *not* be standard." But to respect individuality it must be extracted from the individual: "By recognizing individuality and encouraging its expression we will have a consistency of general approach coupled with a rich variety of person-oriented care plans."[40] And one achieves this coupling of general approach and individualized care through the health care team formed into a support group: "Places which provide opportunities for patients and/or their families to engage in either private conversations or more intimate caring relationships would be a significant beginning. . . . Day rooms that invite conversation with others could also be a place where patients and their families could gain support and understanding from one another." To this environment that "invites" conversation is added the team: "In addition to the attending physician, an interdisciplinary team including a counselor or psychologist, a social worker, a minister, a recreational therapist and a nurse could be specifically designated to respond to the various needs of the dying patient and his family. . . . The team could focus on the 'whole person.' "[41]

Modern medicine has moved away from its former ideal of eliminating death. Now it proposes to serve up the good life climaxed by an appropriate death. Some medical researchers feel that already we are approaching this new ideal. Dr. James Fries of Stanford

believes, for example, that "the medical and social task of eliminating premature death is largely accomplished." In an anticipat-
able scenario, physicians suggest, most of us will live actively for
80 or 90 years and then die quickly but nicely and discreetly from
a severely diminished biological capacity to cope with the slightest
perturbation in the structure of our holon. [42]

It is instructive that the most visible support groups have formed
around birthing and dying. These are, respectively, the point at
which death enters the world and the point at which the awesome
power of death is finally realized. These most "painful" parts of
life have been neutralized and recreated in positive, pleasurable,
ultimately sexual terms by the normalizing technologies of the support group. The support group is a more ubiquitous form, however.
It is the form of the new medical encounter which has been deployed across the entire life span.

The new medical encounter is characterized by virtual equality
of the patient and physician. The physician must not presume to
speak across the gulf of silence that characterized the early practice
of medicine; the physician must now empathize with the patient.
Texts say, ". . . assay the intellectual, emotional, and social capacities of the patient, and pitch the content of the conversation
accordingly. It is important to avoid a patronizing air, whatever the
patient's intellectual level,"[43] and "Empathy is a critical tool in the
interview. The physician attempts to place himself in the patient's
position, to feel what the patient feels, to experience the same
circumstances; if a physician is successful at this, the patient will
feel understood and the physician will have a better idea of how
to be helpful in psychologically supporting the patient."[44] Eventually the physician must discriminate among the features of a
patient's problem and decide which merit primary attention, but
the first goal of the physician is to provide *support,* "the expression
of positive affect of one person toward another; the affirmation or
endorsement of another person's behaviors, perceptions, or expressed views; the giving of symbolic or material aid to another."[45]
The new patient-physician encounter elevates the patient's prob-

lems to a level of principal importance and requires that the doctor acknowledge and affirm the patient as a person. But to what end?

Put simply, medicine aims for an optimal order. The life-span perspective forces medicine to focus on all disruptive and dislocative aspects of life. Disturbances in the relationships within the holon hierarchy of systems are problematic, and medicine's task is to restore order. Birth is disruptive. It disrupts a woman's internal organs, the family, the community, and so forth up and down the holon. Death is disruptive. So are problems of adolescence, early adult life, midlife, and so on. The new medical logic proposes to meet disruption and dislocation with a policy of *"preventive optimization* and not only alleviation"[46] which extends over the entire life course. Such a policy incorporates many of the features of modern medicine mentioned already. It respects the person but does not focus only on the sick person. It does not spring to action only as the sick person enters the clinic seeking cure, but it reaches out, locating the person in the community, anticipating problems before they occur, and making judgments about the optimal use of limited resources to meet a multiplicity of problems. This policy leaves the physician in a privileged position but subordinates him to a higher vision than simply health. The physician as well as the patient become subordinate to a vision of order, a generally healthy order, but not an order necessarily based on health.

Order presumes control, and control usually implies a suppression of individuality. It is by resolving this incompatibility between the problem of order and the emergence of the individual that the sociological beauty and the full power of the support group become fully evident.

Medicine realizes that there is, inherent in its own logic, a tension between the interests or needs of the individual and the interests or needs of social order. "Growth and development involve conflicts between the gratification of one's own instincts, drives, wishes, and needs on the one hand, and, on the other, the wishes, needs, and demands of other people and society," says one text.[47] Or, as another put the problem, "[there is a] seeming absence of a defined

goal for humankind and of a common answer to questions about
life and death and the future. We need to define ourselves as individuals and to find our fates."[48]

The support group, generically speaking, affirms the individual
and simultaneously, effects order, a "fit between the person and
the environment," and an ability to "cope" or adapt to changes
around us. One author divides "support" into three parts: *network*
support, which makes a person feel a part of a community; *esteem*
support, which gives a person a sense of worth; and *emotional*
support, which gives the person a feeling of being cared for and
loved. "Those who are esteemed, therefore self-confident, and those
who are emotionally supported, therefore comfortable, are more
able to change themselves to fit into a changed environment. Similarly, those who are confident have a sense of autonomy and are
more likely to engage in coping behavior, and so are more likely
to take control of their environments and to manipulate those environments into a more acceptable shape. By the same token, Network Support and Esteem Support contribute to a sense of
participation in decision making, which likewise contributes to environmental control, or at least to the 'illusion of control' which
may be as important as actual control."[49] The support group thus
becomes the tie between the individual and a happier, healthier
social order, that which facilitates individual expressivity and simultaneously maintains a smoothly functioning social order not
threatened by individualism. Sidney Cobb, the author of the model
just described, believes that "One cannot escape the conclusion
that the world would be a healthier place if training in supportive
behavior were built into the routines of our homes and schools,
and support worker roles were institutionalized."[50] Cobb has turned
Illich's wry analysis that "Industrialized humanity needs therapy
from crib to terminal ward"[51] into a virtue for which medicine
should aim.

The doctor and the patient join together, then, in the adventure
of life. It is a well mapped adventure with each step well anticipated,
each deviation from the good life monitored, and disruptions in the

hierarchy of systems acted on. It is an adventure whose veridical correspondence to life is confirmed by the good death of every adventurer. Above all, it is an adventure that insures *order,* the order for which Roquentin longed so much. Unfortunately for medicine, though, nothing inherent in the adventure it writes says how the individual is to be enticed to come to accept medicine's vision of order. Individuals might not choose to enter into a joint adventure. How does the new logic address this problem?

## Eight

# Becoming True to Your Own Nature: Victim Blaming and New Social Technologies

IN 1630 AND 1631, plague raged through the Arno River valley near Florence. Monte Lupo, a small, poverty-stricken castello, was particularly hard hit. Off and on during the two-year period, health authorities in Florence called on Father Giovanni Dragoni to administer strict quarantine and policing orders imposed on the city to contain and battle the plague. Surgeons were sent to diagnose and treat the sick. The monastery was seized to serve as a sick house. Records of the living, the dying, and the dead were kept with scrupulous accuracy. Passes for movement in and out of the town were issued. Guards were deployed to keep order. Subsidies were sent to keep the town alive since the quarantine measures suspended all economic activity.

Don Antonio Bontadi, the priest of Monte Lupo, had different ideas about how the plague should be met. On Sunday and Monday, July 20 and 21, 1631, Don Antonio brought the miraculous crucifix of Monte Lupo out of the church, paraded it through the town, and engaged the plague in a battle based on his religious faith. People from nearby villages joined the people of Monte Lupo in the processions, celebrations and ceremonies conducted in defiance of the health authorities. On several occasions the priest confronted the guards sent by the Florentine Health Magistracy, and in every instance the guards decided it was in their best interests to withdraw once they saw the size of the throngs of faithful assembled around the priest.[1]

Dragoni and Don Antonio represented two opposing approaches to controlling the plague. The plague was a signal that the priest's prayerful, meditative life of self-sacrifice practiced behind monastery walls had not succeeded in keeping order in the world, and that God had looked upon the area with particular disfavor. Both Dragoni and Don Antonio came out of the silence of the monastery to contend with the plague, but they assumed two different postures once there. Father Dragoni, without knowing the cause of the epidemic, had his orders. The force of reason buried him behind an elaborate bureaucratic system of surveillance and administration. Dragoni disappeared into a rational, logical apparatus deployed inside the walls of little Monte Lupo. He did not have to adopt this posture and, in fact, he had before him in the person of a fellow priest a model for an alternative form of behavior.

Don Antonio knew, to his satisfaction, the cause of Monte Lupo's woes. Once established, plagues persisted in certain areas, according to priests, because the "city's silence toward God displeased Him," and because of the "blindness of men who think they can remedy this loss of life that is sent from Heaven, solely with human care contrary to the Almighty's purpose."[2] The only possible way to meet the plague, so religious reasoning went, was to tell the townspeople the cause of their problems, engage them in ceremonies of penitence, and get everyone to pray that they should be delivered from disease so that the town could function properly again. While it might be humankind's fate to suffer death because of its location in the universal moral order of things, the fault for the viciousness of death brought by the plague lay with the town. Religion understood that death had a purpose. This understanding derived from Don Antonio's form of logic and reason.

The force of the new medical logic, not unlike the force of reason whose agent was Dragoni, threatens to bury the modern physician in a health care team and a widely deployed health care organization if that logic is allowed to proceed unchecked. The physician will become, at best, a systems manager and, at worst, just another part of a "pool of resources" to be called upon as necessary. The new medical logic is causing the physician to disappear. How medicine responds to this pressure becomes an interesting empirical question. Part of what is happening, we believe, can be likened to Don Antonio's behavior. Medicine is trying to maintain the gulf between the physician and patient across which the physician always spoke with the power of an uninterrupted truth. The new medical logic threatens to bridge the gulf and reshape the field of medical power so that the physician no longer occupies the privileged center. Medicine is trying to resist.

More than 300 years after the events in Monte Lupo, William Ryan, a social psychologist, called Don Antonio's kind of thinking "blaming the victim." The town suffers disease and pestilence as anything in the secular world can be expected to, but the blame for *this* disease and the continuation of disease as severe as *this* one must lie with the victim, the town in this case. If only the victim could be different—if only the town would pray harder, pull itself out of its poverty, live the life it knows it should—it would not suffer to such an extent. In piety and desperation Don Antonio drew out the crucifix and marched it through the town, trying to excise the plague just as the surgeon plunges a scalpel into the body of a patient hoping to excise a disease and prevent a death that, were it but for the chosen behavior of the patient, would never have appeared in the first place. This time the effort may succeed, but hope for the future can only rest on a change in the way the patient—the town or the diseased person—lives its life. Viewed from across the gulf of a privileged knowledge, the victim gets blamed for living his life badly.

As Ryan described the practice, blaming the victim "shifts its emphasis to the environmental causation" of problems and away from genetic or other causes inherent to the victim, but the blame for falling prey to problems still rests with the victim. "The stigma that marks the victim and accounts for his victimization is an acquired stigma, a stigma of social rather than genetic origin. But," says Ryan, "the stigma, the defect, the fatal difference—though derived in the past from environmental forces—is still located *within* the victim, inside his skin."[3] Once a problem is located in this way, the path toward change is clear: "Prescriptions for cure . . . are invariably conceived to revamp and revise the victim, never to change the surrounding circumstances. They want to change his attitudes, alter his values, fill up his cultural deficits, energize his apathetic soul, cure his character defects, train him and polish him and woo him from his savage ways."[4]

We can see why the victim-blaming approach has been so attractive to medicine. The first step one has to take in order to blame the victim—noting environmental causes of social and individual ills—allows one to appear to adopt an ecological perspective on a problem. The cause of failure or disease is not something buried in the afflicted individual and therefore unapproachable and immutable; instead, causal forces are located outside the individual and, therefore, are changeable in principle. But changing an environment and thereby changing the underlying causes of all ills is difficult. At best, it is a long-term project. In the short term other avenues for remedy are possible, and to the physician they are immediately accessible. The physician can ask, what is it about this person that makes him/her so vulnerable to environmental causes of problems? Treatment can still be directed at the individual patient. Failure to construct management schemes aimed primarily at the environment can be easily rationalized. Victim-blaming logic allows medicine tentatively to embrace some of the implications of an ecological perspective and systems-theoretic logic without having to follow that logic to its furthest points.

Blaming the victim has another advantage that fits well into traditional medical thinking. It can be done with dispassionate, unemotional objectivity; it can be done from behind the security of the monastery wall. Humanitarian, liberal reformers find victims of social problems and then try to reform them as individuals. "They want to make the victims less vulnerable, send them as individuals back into battle with better weapons, thicker armor, a higher level of morale." But, "In order to do so effectively—they must analyze the victims carefully, dispassionately, objectively, scientifically, emphatically, mathematically, and hardheadedly, to see what made them so vulnerable in the first place."[5] Appeals to victim blaming allow medicine to eliminate the confounding influences of the emotionalism of everyday life so that those influences do not confuse the assessor and lead to an incorrect diagnosis. This was what medicine had done for nearly two centuries. Like the priest who may leave the monastery only with crucifix in hand and only to excise the plague, like the priest who must not venture into the town and dirty his hands in the day-to-day commerce and life of the city, the traditional physician did not enter into the lives of his patients. Patients were taken out of life, brought into the neutral domain of the clinic, and subjected to that informed gaze that sees beyond them into the truth of disease and death. Blaming the victim permits the physician to maintain an old posture and to analyze and judge his patient while he himself remains on neutral ground, unanalyzed, and above all, unjudged even by, perhaps particularly by, himself.

Victim blaming appears in many corners of medical discourse. The "defaulter" who engages in "non-compliance" with prescribed therapeutic regimens caught medicine's attention just prior to 1940, and from the recognition that a patient might choose not to follow doctor's orders sprang the thriving field of compliance research. Researchers recognized early that environmental factors—whether a therapeutic regimen required a change in daily routines or perhaps a change of jobs, whether someone took an interest in the patient's compliance, the number of pills a person had to take, the physical characteristics of the pills and the ease with which one pill could be distinguished from another—influenced compliance significantly. Still, their research directed attention toward the patient, his or her personality and beliefs about an illness or about health and toward education designed to overcome any barriers to compliance that might be found in the patient. So, for example, as late as 1973, a review article emphasized the influence of personality traits on compliance: "[Patients] with poorest compliance [in a study of psychiatric outpatients] showed the greatest degree of hostility and aggression''; ''Women who fail to take their contraceptive pills regularly have been found to be more immature, irresponsible, and impulsive''; ''At the same time there are other personality types who may be reluctant to take medication for different reasons. These include the obsessional with fears of losing control or becoming drug dependent or who simply wishes to 'do it alone.' Finally, there are the paranoid or hypochondriacal patients who fear that medication may harm them.''[6]

Personality characteristics mediated beliefs about a disease, medicine thought, and it was toward those causally prior ''health beliefs'' that education programs were directed to alter the patient and improve compliance: ''Even before prescribing it is important for the patient to understand the illness and its probable duration or consequences so that treatment appears logical and necessary.''[7] In effect, the patient who insists on acting healthy must be changed and made to believe that he is not.

Presently, victim blaming is more evident on larger scales than it is at the individual level. At the level of analysis of whole health care systems, victim blaming becomes a political strategy for directing attention away from the social causes of social problems and toward the individual causes of social problems. Lifestyle is the real problem, victim blaming tells us, not the dangers of the workplace, the pollutants pumped into the environment, or the additives put into foods. If lifestyle is the problem, the individual can be called to account for his own difficulties while others, those who created dangerous environments in the first place, are tacitly absolved of responsibility. While the federal government decides whether or not to accept responsibility for increased lung cancer rates among people who worked with asbestos in shipyards during World War II, the workers are admonished not to smoke because smoking increases their risk of lung cancer four times over fellow workers who do not smoke. Despite a federal government report indicating that heart disease would be reduced by only 25% if individual, ''lifestyle'' factors including cholesterol level, smoking, blood sugar levels, blood pressure, serum uric acid level and so on were perfectly controlled,[8] research still focuses on correlations of personality traits with heart disease. Recently for example, the National Institutes of Health funded a five-year study of the effects of Type A behavior on heart attacks. Type A behavior is a complex of personality traits thought to be associated with heart attacks. The Type A person has a strong achievement orientation, is competitive, impatient, aggressive, and has a strong commitment to work. The NIH-sponsored study is designed to see if changing one's "stressful" way of life will decrease the chances of second heart attacks among the study's 900 subjects who have had one heart attack already. According to James Gill, a researcher on the project, changing one's behavior in fact reduces the chance of coronary care unit recidivism. "In every instance of a recurrence we can recall, the individual had violated the advice" of his physician, Gill told the *New York Times*.[9]

Medicine brings heart attack victims into its labs, assesses their Type A personality score, encourages them to discuss their lifestyle problems in therapeutic groups, and teaches them exercises for changing behavior and attitudes. Then medicine sends them out of the lab, back into the environment which encourages and rewards a high achievement orientation, competitiveness, aggressiveness, and a strong commitment to work, and later, if they have another heart attack, medicine blames them for not following doctor's orders. The environment, the economic system, the workplace, the day-to-day pressures of modern life go relatively unconsidered and absolutely untouched.

In the mid-1970s several influential books promulgated a victim-blaming ideology, and important people in the health policy field adopted the ideology as a rallying point for medical reform. Three critical analyses of modern medicine published during the period helped foster the notion that individuals, not medicine, had to be responsible for the health of the nation. Ivan Illich's book *Medical Nemesis*[10] claimed that the health care systems of advanced countries like the United States are iatrogenic; that is, Illich felt the systems themselves cause disease. Appearing in 1976, just as the cost-containment critique of medicine was beginning to boil, Illich's calls for "deinstitutionalizing" medicine received a warm hearing in various sectors of the very establishment Illich wanted to criticize. Cutbacks were inevitable, and ironically Illich provided a rationale for them. At about the same time Rick Carlson argued for individualistic, seemingly metaphysical alternatives to scientific medicine in his book *The End of Medicine*.[11] After his wide-ranging critique of modern medicine, Carlson recommended without any critical reflection at all that we adopt the techniques of acupuncture, para-psychology, psychic surgery, and the like to solve many of the nation's health problems.

Illich's and Carlson's books complemented positions set forward in the 1974 book by Victor R. Fuchs, *Who Shall Live?*[12] According to Fuchs, all health problems have a basis in individual choices. "The oft-heard statement, 'Health is the most important goal,' does not accurately describe human behavior. Every day in manifold ways (such as overeating or smoking) we make choices that affect our health, and it is clear that we frequently place a higher value on satisfying other wants."[13] Fuchs is aware of many of the "environmental causes" of disease, and most of his recommendations for change are macrosocial and systemic in nature. But in his penultimate position statement he vitiates the possibility of the truly radical, systemic change that his analysis would seem to require. The fundamental problem impeding reform, Fuchs argues, is the problem of "value choices," choices about the kind of society we live in and want to have in the future. Making choices that lead to continued tolerance of inequality is at the heart of our problems. "The problem of inequality should be faced head on," Fuchs says, adding the crucial caveat: *"in ways that do the least damage to the efficient performance of the economy."*[14]

A victim-blaming argument flows freely from this position since it does not allow that it may be the economy that requires and fosters the inequality of which Fuchs is so critical. If we cannot change the economy substantially, we must change people's unhealthy behavior in it. His book closes with the following claim:

"By changing institutions and creating new programs we can make medical care more accessible and deliver it more efficiently but the greatest potential for improving health lies in what we do and don't do for and to ourselves. The choice is ours."[15]

For Fuchs, changes in lifestyle are the only possible answer to the most serious health problems faced by modern society. He believes that lifestyle is a matter of choice for most people in the modern world, whereas, to a large degree, lifestyle is an adaptation to social and economic conditions over which most people have only the smallest degree of control. Fuchs, along with Illich and Carlson, believes that individuals must be responsible for health now because the institution to which we collectively ceded responsibility a century earlier has proven itself ineffective. It is rather bold to assume individuals can effectively take responsibility for their own health. Ironically perhaps, it is also rather conservative to assume so because, as Howard Berliner has argued, "Discussing changes in lifestyles without first discussing the changes in the social conditions which give rise to them, without recognizing that the lifestyle is derivative, is misleading and, in effect, victim blaming."[16]

Victim blaming diffused throughout the medical policy-making apparatus quickly in the 1970s. While president of the Rockefeller Foundation, John Knowles said, "One man's or woman's freedom in health is now another man's shackle in taxes and insurance premiums. . . . The choice is, in fact, over the long range individual responsibility or social failure."[17] Knowles was preemptively blaming the individual for our collective demise. Similarly the president of Blue Cross, dismayed by the modern search for the quick technological fix, said, "People must have the capability and the will to take greater responsibility for their own health."[18] By living better the individual can do good for himself/herself and for the country. This was the message that policy makers sent out.

Victim blaming is still around. It is a politically effective form of reasoning, but, as we said earlier, whether medicine first adopts and then holds onto a victim-blaming stance or not are empirical questions. Medicine did adopt such a posture for a decade or so, and we have outlined some of the ways victim blaming appeared in medicine. Now, however, it appears that a different approach is gaining ascendancy. Medicine seems to be following its own new logic where the logic leads.

Medicine is changing so that its work looks more like the work of the health authorities in Monte Lupo, personified by Father Dragoni, than like the work of the castello priest. Instead of meeting the plague with a crucifix, a ceremony, and prayers that the plague be taken away, the Health Board of Florence met the plague with instructions for dividing up the city; for isolating all individuals—the sick and the healthy—one from the other; for monitoring all movement into, out of, and within the town; for diagnosing disease, burying the dead, feeding the quarantined; and for keeping records on everything that happened in the town.[19] Without knowing the "true" causes of the disease or the vectors by which it was transmitted, they fought it with what Foucault has called "an organization in depth of surveillance and control, an intensification and a ramification of power"[20] designed first to analyze the idiosyncratic relationships and dynamics of the town and second to control them in the hope of controlling the disease.

After 1950, medicine reoriented itself to pay attention to the idiosyncracies of patients and to the relationships patients had with other parts of the environment. Specialties continued to multiply, but they were tied together under comprehensive views of disease and doctoring. Knowing and analyzing became almost more important than acting, and prevention superseded intervention. As medicine adopted an ecological orientation, the surgeon who approached the silent patient in a priestly fashion gave way to the family practice specialist surrounded by a well integrated array of other specialists who approached disease with a new kind of "watchful and armed expectancy," much as a prison guard, knowing that his own future is tied to the orderly operation of the prison, watches every movement carefully and listens closely for the faintest, most distant sign of disharmony.

The moralistic and moralizing approach of victim blaming is uncharacteristic of the modern expert of whom Donzelot wrote. A moral discourse is the basis for a form of power that excludes. Sociologists have long understood that society must invent concepts of deviance in order to establish and maintain social boundaries that delimit for a social group what its members are to value as real and true about their conduct. Concepts of deviance demonstrate the existence of boundaries by placing some people on the outside of them in opposition to the social group. Sociologists have tended to understand such concepts as central to the practices of power. This was, for example, the function of the scarlet letter worn by Hester Prynne. She was a public demonstration of the immoral, a person left alone by the force of power to walk the streets with her infant and her letter. Foucault, however, has tried to show that to focus on exclusionary practices which surround concepts of deviance provides a limited, if not essentially incorrect understanding of power.[21]

Modern practices of power, explicitly those that operate in medicine, are not organized on the basis of a moral discourse about persons, but on the basis of a possibility, born in the nineteenth century, of conducting a scientific-technical discourse on the individual. The ultimate expression of power in a moral discourse is exclusion. To be cast into a dark and confused space where one has no place and where one is constantly surrounded by the horrible possibilities of the unknown is moral power's threatening face. Fear of exclusion maintains order as power fashions itself as a ubiquitous, if at times unseen, police force.

Modern power operates through inclusion, not exclusion. Power that illuminates, analyzes and grasps its object is more effective than power that leaves its object alone, even though "alone" means life in a darkened space beyond the limits of the accepted and the acceptable. Modern power erases moral oppositions and redefines them as differentiated, encapsulated units within the limits of the social. The scientific discourse about the inidividual invents the individual as an object to be measured and managed in a social space that no longer has a boundary since it incorporates everything in the name of seeking "scientific truth."

Of all the types of scientific discourse about the individual the most recent is the discourse on sexual desire. It is certainly the most significant incursion into the domain of subjectivity, the private and concealed domain which traditionally undergirded one's "individuality." Part of this discourse focuses on a problem that recently became a "medical problem": teenage pregnancy. "Teenage pregnancy" is a concept that appeared for the first time in the late 1960s. It is the scientific analog of the moralistic categories of "unwed mother" and "illegitimate child." By investigating the appearance of this new idea we can begin to appreciate the modern practice of power that is inclusionary.

The subjective experience of sexual desire is a danger that becomes a social threat since desire can aim at any object. A society organized on the basis of a moral discourse meets this threat by socially separating the aims of sexual desire from its objects. Once aims and objects of desire are separated, society can define the "right objects" for desire to aim at. "Right objects" create their own, moral opposites: perversions, including perverse maternity. The subjective experience of sexual desire traditionally was placed under the superintendency of the law that punished perversions like "unwed mothers" who had "illegitimate children." A moral discourse makes sexual desire a subjective freedom that is subject to punishment, often harsh punishment, under law, but that is inviolable to knowledge.

A scientific discourse, on the other hand, is concerned with the total truth of an individual, including the truth of one's sexual desires. It defines an individual's sexual desires in terms of the objects it aims at. The truth of desire under a scientific discourse is not that desire is free to choose its own objects (as it is under a moral discourse), but, conversely, the object desire aims at creates the truth of desire, which is available as an object of "expert" knowledge. The scientific discourse is a language of taxonomies and "types" of desire. Each type is defined by the object desire aims at. The scientific discourse on the individual, by its own rules, begins with a degraded subjectivity, which is not free (though it is subject to punishment) but is, instead, to be known, analyzed, discussed, and managed.

The scientific discourse does not dispose of notions of sexual deviance. It simply invents a new kind of deviance based on the "fact" that desire does not always conform to its own truth. The sexual deviant is one who is in error about his or her sexual desire, one who is not true to his or her own nature. Fortunately, we say, the truth of sexual desire is known to an "expert" whose function it is to practice truth on desires that are "errors" that can be "corrected." People can become true to their own natures, natures that are determined to be true by the experts.

The focus of the *moral* problem of adolescent pregnancy was the mother. She represented the danger of unbridled, rampant sexuality. Her sexuality was portrayed as the dark side of life, a kind of animal freedom. The child was not of great interest. The child was an object of compassion, while at the same time it served as a badge of the mother's immorality.

In 1943, teenage sexuality created "trouble on the street corners." It was the middle of the Second World War, and "these 'victory girls' and 'cuddle bunnies' who go uniform hunting in railroad stations and wander down Main Street late at night looking for pick ups are just ordinary kids who have been swept along in a torrent of wartime excitement and free spending."[22] Such wild women "swell[ed] the venereal disease rate as tragically as if they were hardened professionals" and caused illegitimacy rates to soar.[23] A surgeon general of an air base reportedly said, "Good-time girls of high school age are the army's biggest potential source of venereal disease."[24]

The real problem was that the whole problem was not obeying class lines. " 'It's the good girls who get into trouble,' a social worker said. 'The bad ones know how to avoid it.' "[25] The Florence Crittenden League, one of the earliest organizations for unwed mothers, reported in the early 1940s that more of its clients were coming from "respectable homes."[26] So the increase in problems associated with adolescent sexuality could not be attributed to the bad, if perhaps "understandable," behavior of women of the lower classes or to increases in the ranks of "hardened professionals." Something more was going on. Whatever the causes, more and more women were transgressing moral laws; they were finding themselves on the outside of society, wandering, lost, and excluded.

The imagery of exclusion permeates the popular literature on teenage sexuality from the forties through the early sixties. This was a period of dichotomies in sexuality: right-wrong, moral-immoral, inside-outside, human-animal. In June 1948, the *Reader's Digest* published a symposium called, "Must we change our sex standards?" to which J. Edgar Hoover, the preeminent moralist of the time, contributed this: "Whenever the American people, young or old, come to believe that there is no such thing as right or wrong, normal or abnormal, those who would destroy our civilization will applaud a major victory over our way of life."[27] In an article recommending community financial aid for those people who wished to marry young, Will C. Turnbladh of the National Probation Association accounted for the facts that communities were "up to their necks in delinquency" and that "the number of wayward girls, young sex offenders, and unmarried mothers" was increasing by arguing that young people were up against a "stone wall."[28] In 1963, an author said of the practice of referring to women in homes for unwed mothers by their first names and last initials, "While this anonymity is merciful, it is also symptomatic of the way we treat illegitimacy in this country: by isolating the offender. . . . Whatever a girl's story, there is no question about society's response to her plight: it ostracizes her."[29]

There was always, during this period, a concern for preventing transgressions, a concern about society's responsibility to help people behave in the right way. Finding right actions for youth—right objects for desire—was often offered as the ultimate solution to the problems of unwed mothers, illegitimate children and the like: "[One solution] goes further toward the root of the problem. It is

to give forgotten, restless girls the right kind of wartime responsibility and the right kind of adolescent fun."[30] "The case for making
marriage available to hundreds of thousands of the blocked generation is not built on sentiment: it is a serious business of saving
young people from frustration, of preserving the American home,
of stemming the tidal waves of promiscuity, delinquency and di-
vorce."[31] Marriage or at least appropriate fun, not animal sexuality
outside marriage, was the right object for sexual desire to aim at.

In the early sixties pregnant adolescents who were public demonstrations of the existence of a moral order gained a degree of
publicity that began to invoke more seriously than ever before the
idea of rehabilitation. Medicalization of adolescent sexuality (but
"medicalization" of a sort different from that which followed the
"look into the body and see" rule of traditional medicine) moved
the problem away from its moral locus. "Doctors and social workers," wrote one person in 1963, "are just now beginning to put
some of their best efforts into rehabilitation. At some of the Salvation Army maternity homes, there is a growing push behind the
'after care' program, designed to keep a troubled girl in contact
with her social workers during the reintegration period. . . ."[32] Then
in the late sixties a number of articles appeared publicly exposing
for the first time what had been spoken of only in the most coded
language of moral separations.

The first article to show pictures of pregnant teens—unwed moth-
ers-to-be—appeared in 1966 in *Ebony*.[33] Pictures in articles like this
one are ideographic. That is, they are "graphic illustrations of
certain ideas . . . and not purely 'true to nature,'"[34] or "matter of
fact." The picture that appears under the title of the *Ebony* article
shows a physician taking a young woman's blood pressure. The
doctor looks at his instrument. The girl's eyes are photographically
masked so that we see no identifying features. Behind the physician
is a nurse who smiles broadly at two babies in her arms. This picture
carries the dual message prevalent at the end of the period when
teenage pregnancy was a moral problem handled through the techniques of exclusion. First, the teen and her child are subject to two

types of care: the nurse shows obvious joy over the babies; the doctor shows an indifferent concern for the mother. The teenage mother is an object of medical concern and is not simply a person who demonstrates the existence of a sociomoral boundary by her presence on the other side of it. Her baby, previously an outward symbol of the mother's transgression, is now a source of value. Yet—and this is the second message—the mother has become invisible. She has no face of her own. Her identity is barred from surfacing. She is effaced (literally) by the sudden visibility of the infant who is depicted as an object of value, i.e., a joy, a treasure.

The significance of the sudden visibility of the child does not lie in a "discovery" of the child. He or she was always present and visible. The child was an innocent object of compassion, a product of the mother's misdeeds. The significance of the child's visibility lies instead in the effacement of the mother. Her disappearance supplies the context for the child's brilliant presence. Casting the mother into the shadows at the same time the child achieves a shining new status poses a problem and a question: "We cannot speak of someone who produces such a treasure as this child as sinful and immoral. What then are we to say of this woman?" The mother seems to have been excluded from the picture, but she is not simply excluded, for she is, for the first time, visible. She has been removed to a position where she no longer has to be a living testimony to her own sinfulness. She no longer represents transgression, animality, or "otherness." Indeed, she has been neutralized and seems to represent nothing. But no thing can represent nothing. Consequently, she incites us to a discourse about her since she no longer represents either herself or the Other. Her "disappearance" is less a placing of the pregnant woman under a taboo than an incitement to discourse of the sort Foucault talks about in his analysis of the Victorian taboo on sex.[35] We are left with our question: "What must we say about her given that something must be said?" This is the stage just prior to the invention of "teenage pregnancy" as a "fact of knowledge."

Pregnant teens turned around and had their faces unmasked in

1971. The pregnant adolescent reappears as the teenage mother. She is no longer an effaced, neutralized being, but she reappears in the context of a neutralized sexuality. Sexuality's truth lies not in morality but instead in biology. Perhaps its truth lies not even in biology as much as in the biopsycho-social complex of the holon. The pregnant teen becomes simply an error, a deviation from proper placement of sexuality and sexual desire in a sequenced and hierarchical set of reproductive subsystems. Sexuality occurs in accordance with the scientifically lawful knowledge we have about the "true place"[36] of human sexuality and reproduction in the social order.

In 1971, *Life* magazine[37] showed on its cover a picture of a young woman in the late stages of pregnancy reading to her high school class. In the *Life* article pregnant teens are no longer excluded. They are no longer an anonymous part of an undifferentiated mass allowed to exist in a place specially provided for them. They are individuals who belong. They are part of the high school crowd. The woman on the cover is shown inside the magazine smiling and joking with her friends. Teenage mothers are different but they are included. When they are shown receiving childcare instructions along with other pregnant teens and unwed mothers, half of them face the camera and half of them face away. The person who instructs is no longer the central figure in these ideographs. Pregnant teens gain a visibility they had not had before. One teen's words, bannered across a picture in the middle of the *Life* story, declare the essence of the change that took place very quickly during the early seventies. She says, "I feel like a person again."

A moral problem rests on division. In the case of teenage pregnancy the division was between "personhood" and "nonpersonhood." Once teens could declare, "I feel like a person again," the conceptual infrastructure for treating teenage pregnancy as a moral problem disappeared. A September 1948 article foretold the course that teenage pregnancy would follow: "[Courses in sex education] are adding still more facts to the topheavy load on a foundation in which the moral cement is crumbling."[38] Knowledge destroys the capacity for morality, the author seems to be saying, unless of course the moral laws are so strong that they can withstand the heavy burden of facts. "Without definite, as well as general, moral laws, facts are destructive and moral authority is impossible."[39] Throughout the sixties and early seventies we would come to know more about teenage pregnancy—we would become more familiar with pregnant teenage women and see their faces—and, in fact, a moral response to the pregnant teen would become impossible. The basis of authority would shift and teenage pregnancy would become a technical problem.

A moral law removes a phenomenon to a place where the existence of the phenomenon is known but the details of the phenomenon can be ignored. Knowledge of the immoral is complete once we know it is wrong. Details become titillating, suggestive, occasionally seductive, but they remain forbidden. On the other hand, a phenomenon that is a technical problem does more than simply allow knowledge of its details; a technical problem compels analysis and requires detailed knowledge of its fine structure.

Sexual desire is no longer a dangerous force which can aim perversely at perverse objects. It has gained a passivity by gaining a new "nature" as one component in a system whose natural aim is a balanced harmony. The question to be asked today is not, "How are we to discover and punish desire that aims at perverse objects in its dark and concealed actions?" but, instead, "Why is sexual desire not in its proper place in the balanced order of things? What has caused desire's aim to be in error?" Moral rules used to exclude; one might be inside moral laws or outside them. Now everyone lives on the inside since the "essence of morality"[40] lies in a technical truth about life as a system whose components strive for integration and coordination, a "natural" balance and harmony.

In 1981 the Alan Guttmacher Institute published a compendium of facts about teenage pregnancy called, "Teenage Pregnancy: The Problem that Hasn't Gone Away."[41] It is important not so much for what it tells us about teenage pregnancy as for the way it says what it says. In the same way the pictures in *Ebony* carried a double message of joy over the babies and indifference to the mother, the pictures in the Guttmacher Institute pamphlet also carry a double message but of a different sort. The bottom half of the pamphlet's cover is a grid—graph paper. The lower halves of most of the pages in the book are filled with graphs and maps—the facts of what is known about this technical problem that hasn't gone away. The first message is clear enough, then: we know a lot, maybe not enough, and we can always know more, better, in greater detail.

The second message is a little more muted. Embedded in the grid on the cover is a picture of a woman with a baby. The woman is visible and knowable, individually and as a member of an epidemiological category. Yet in this picture there is no clear expression of joy over the baby, which the nurse demonstrated so clearly in the *Ebony* article. The picture suggests that this woman might be deeply and romantically in love with the baby, but then, as we study the picture more, its character changes and the woman appears close to her baby but rather indifferent to it. She may be kissing the child or checking to see if it has vomited. The emotionality in the picture is ambiguous and mirrors what the experts tell us about the conflicted lability of adolescent emotion. Mother and child are presented in terms of what we know according to a grid that maps the location and movement of an individual life.

Mapping and charting life extend even to a woman's emotionality, the last refuge of subjectivity. We know what is true about the depth and range of the emotionality of adolescent girls. After all, the experts on human development have mapped it for us! It is true that "Teenage Pregnancy" contains pictures that show joy and laughter, but teenage boys and girls laugh only when they are located in their age group doing what is proper to the truth of their teenage nature. Teens smile broadly as they read together a book on love. Girls laugh girlishly at diaphragm fitting sessions. Girls even laugh girlishly at their friend's round stomach which is a sign of an error to which desire is prone when its aim is not true to nature. But no one laughs at babies. Women scream during labor. They manage a somber smile when they are alone and pregnant.

They strike a subdued pose as a family of teenage parents with a new baby. They hug babies close. One woman smiles slightly when a baby pulls her hair. But no one laughs.

The concept "teenage pregnancy" as an "error" has appeared and with it has come a new concept of care. Care now requires management of an error as if it were a technical problem. Management requires, first, a visible issue or concern and, second, the determination of a proper balance among conflicting aspects of the issue or a proper path through the maze that the issue presents. The technical problem of teenage pregnancy has both.

Teenage pregnancy is not just visible in the pictures in national publications; pregnant teens have become visible and knowable as individuals. An article in *The PTA Magazine* in 1970 began with a personal description of "Joanne," black, pregnant in high school, and at the time of the article an honor student in college. She was a "symbol of a basic—and healthful—change,"[42] but, more important, she was an identifiable individual with friends, feelings and a future. Similarly, a 1972 article in *Today's Health* described in careful detail Fay Ordway, a woman who fought in court to remain in school once she became pregnant. She was "petite and pretty," "star of two class plays . . . anything but a rebel," the article said. She was simply a teenager, knowable as a teenager who possesses the attributes proper to the truth of a teenager—a dependent desire to be educated, a fresh, innocent naiveté about a budding beauty— who happened to become pregnant.[43] Teenage pregnancy was not just a notion that gained visibility through symbolic and rhetorical representation; it was an issue that had a human face produced by the possibility of holding a scientific discourse on the individual.

At about the same time, the notion emerged that there is a proper path for development that would allow one to avoid the problem of teenage pregnancy. "One study of college students revealed that the people who had progressed the most in personality development had a history of gradually unfolding sexual interests and behavior. In other words, their sexual development proceeded at a pace that allowed time for social, emotional and intellectual development," one article said.[44] Proper pace through a correct trajectory establishes a healthy balance is the message. The perspective that admits consideration of teenage pregnancy only as a technical problem is so pervasive that even studies which show, for example, that there is a biological advantage to having children early in life[45] can be dismissed for failing to take into consideration the problem of "balancing" one's life. An editorial in the *American Journal of Public Health* said, "It is not the biological aspect of age that is relevant in our society; it is the social significance. In some other time and place sexual intercourse leading to early reproduction might not be a problem; it might even be an advantage. However, early reproduction in our society has a contemporary disadvantage, the result of modern life."[46] Technical problems invite technological solutions at different levels: "We must continue our efforts to defer the first birth and to improve the social context of reproduction for all our young people."[47]

But how does one create the discipline necessary to achieve such ends? The literature on teenage pregnancy suggests that it is the visibility of teenage pregnancy that creates the discipline required to manage, if not solve, the problem. "Traditionally, U.S. schools have felt that a pregnant girl should be expelled. . . . But the logic of this policy is poor. . . . A single pregnant schoolgirl in study hall—ungainly, unhappy, she and the boy facing responsibilities or hard decisions affecting the rest of their lives—is more eloquent than six sex lectures."[48] Atlanta allowed pregnant teens to continue regular high school classes because it could not afford special education programs for them. This decision, complemented with decisions to provide hospital services and birth control information, "significantly lowered repeat pregnancies, while sharply increasing the number of girls who continued in school, after childbirth, to receive their diplomas."[49] Visibility of a problem reflects back on the problem to become the problem's own disciplining mechanism. Simply recognizing a problem, ironically, may serve as a basis for its solution.

New technologies of division and analysis are operative in teenage pregnancy. The birth of the teenager's baby has been stripped of its negative, moral connotations by treating pregnancy as an event produced by objective forces—biological and social—that can be isolated, differentiated, analyzed and correlated. Of course, the forces that produce life, with all its complexity, are prone to error. Pregnancy is no longer the product of that fathomless emotionality of desire that, as we have always known, aims to unify, meld, fuse and dissolve distinctions. This archaic language of sexual desire has been relegated to a kind of scrap heap of imaginative ruminations suitable for anything but speaking true. Instead of telling of desire that fuses and joins, contemporary ideograms depicting teenage pregnancy are ambiguous about the closeness of mothers and their babies. Laughter and positive emotion are allowed in pictures of boys and girls together where there is absolutely no chance that the obvious, gender-based differences between the actors will collapse. Joy is allowed in pictures of pregnant teens and their non-pregnant friends where, again, the self-evident division between actors will maintain itself. But in pictures of mothers and babies, where the division is conceptually less substantial, strong emotions which threaten to join together the two actors into a single unit are eliminated.

The moves to bring teenage pregnancy out of the shadows, to remove it from a place where it had the ominous, shadowy character of a dark freedom that could go by the name of "trouble on the street corners" and to place it in the full light of day may be just exactly what is required in order to subject the problem to a new form of discipline, management and control, a new operation of power. We are no longer capable of speaking about the teenager in the mixed language of revulsion and envy through which Hawthorne clearly understood the sexual miscreant. We are compelled, it seems, to speak about her instead in the emotionally neutral language of the scientific expert. We treat adolescent pregnancy as an "error" in the proper timing and location of sexual desire. We do not punish the pregnant teen in the old and cruel sense of that word, but instead we are called upon to discipline her to become

"true" to her own "nature," a "nature" the experts have determined to be "true."

To see how new social technologies that discipline one to become
true to one's nature have insinuated themselves into the dying
process consider the report of a dying person. Ted Rosenthal, a
poet with leukemia, writes of the freedom he felt his imminent
death accorded him: "I realized in fact that I felt really good for
the first time in my life. Not just a flash of good feeling, but a
sustained feeling that I had nothing and having nothing, I had nothing to lose, and having nothing to lose I could be anything. I didn't
have a self-image to worry about. And not having a self-image to
worry about meant I had no definition. I had nothing I had to be,
nothing I had to care about. And I felt free. I felt as if I could leap
out the window, not out of despair or fear, but just for the hell of
it, just for the fun of it."[50]

Rosenthal was not living in the sixteenth century where he might
enjoy the freedom to "be anything" even though he would have
been punished severely for not following the moral rules of the
*artes moriendi*. Rosenthal was dying a modern death under a new
practice of power that penetrates even the freedom that imminent
death brings. He writes, "All those people who say that you are
predictable and that you will die in the same way that everyone
else dies, they are right. I resented that at first. I resented them
saying, 'Oh, you are at the two week stage. You're feeling this,
doing this. You're free. You're at the angry stage. I understand
that. You're depressed. You're lost. Three and one half weeks after
you find this out you always feel lost. Well, they're right. It works
that way with me. I'm following patterns. I am following the guide-
lines for dying-of-terminal-cancer patients down to the letter. They
all told me how this would be, how I would be reacting. It's fiendish.
No matter what I say, they say, 'Hm. That's what we thought you'd
say.' "[51] He tells us how he eventually became frightened: "My
medical condition was such that it changed dramatically from moment to moment. . . . I was never able to synchronize my feeling
with information that [came from blood tests and bone marrow

samples], and every bit of information had to alter my feelings about myself in terms of survival and where I stood in relation to the future and even that moment. I became frightened."[52] This man, who could imagine himself leaping from a window for no good reason, is frightened by a distinctly modern experience: not being able to align your subjectivity with the object medicine creates you to be. Eventually, this man who could imagine himself to be anything became just exactly what he was: a dying poet who writes poetically about his dying. He became true to his own nature. It's fiendish, but perhaps we can understand that.

Under the rules of the regime of power that created what Ariès called the era of the tame death, a heavy-handed moral discourse taught the dying what they ought to desire. Yet there remained the implicit freedom desire possesses to roam across an unlimited range of objects, a freedom to "be anything." This freedom was the dark underside of insistent efforts to direct desire toward correct objects, to get the dying to die well. If the dying deviated from the prescribed order, they suffered severe consequences, but they understood this. Their every utterance was attended closely because every utterance had to be rewarded for indicating correct behavior or punished for indicating deviations from correct behavior. Under the new rules of dying, every utterance must be monitored for what it might indicate about the needs of the dying person, not for what it might indicate about their desires. The dying do not enjoy that implicit freedom to oppose themselves to the social, morally correct order of things; they are free only to be different from what they are. They are free only to live erroneously. They can only be deviations from optimal life course trajectories. Utterances reflect a person's deviations back to the person, and the mirror that does the reflecting is the expertly stated, "I understand that." There is no statement the dying can make that cannot be met with this simple yet exceptionally effective disciplinary mechanism. No matter how much a person wishes to escape being what he is, he will be met with total understanding, an understanding that compels alignment with the true nature which the expert understands. It is like Graham Greene's

"Burnt Out Case," a religious architect who retired to a leper colony to live out a life of nothingness. Once news of his rebuilding a small church in the colony was broadcast by the media, he was remade into what he was—a designer of sacred places. Even in a place of absolute exclusion—a leper colony—we are disciplined to be true to our own nature and to become what we are.

Victim blaming was and is an assertion of traditional forms of medicine against a new, more powerful image. It reconstructed in a new milieu crucial elements of a medicine whose logo was the anatomy lesson: the capacity to judge without being judged, the dyad in which only one voice—the voice of "doctor's orders"—speaks and in which the voice of the patient is muted. Victim blaming permitted the physician to resist the force of a logic that would seemingly banish him by converting him into a Father Dragoni, a priest without a parish who serves a form of Reason whose locus is the experts who monitor from a distance. But new technologies which subject the patient to new forms of discipline are apparent in medicine, and resistance to the force of the new logic has become a moot question for how can one resist compassionate, expert understanding?

There is one question that remains. The patient is being made a partner in a joint adventure, the goal of which is to insure order. Unfortunately, nothing in the new logic of medicine specifies the nature of the order the adventure is supposed to insure. Medicine still faces the question, "To what shall we look for a model for order?"

# Nine

# The Vision of Order:
# Ethics, Sociobiology, Spirituality

THE LOGIC OF MODERN medicine forces the physician to serve two masters: the individual and the larger order. An individual who has unrestricted access to the "commons" of health care resources may engage in behavior threatening to the social order as a whole. Physicians today are sometimes called upon to act in ways inimical to the interests of patients in order to protect and preserve the order of the holon. Physicians feel cross-pressured by the logic with which they now must live. John F. Burnam wrote in the *New England Journal of Medicine,* "Ideal medical care depends to an important degree on the physician's being an advocate of the patient. In fact, however, we physicians have long been double agents, serving other interests as well; and now as medical-care rationing begins, we face the unpleasant prospect of representing the conflicting interests of the patient and society."[1] The physician who performs physical examinations for employment purposes or for insurance companies may help the patient by detecting a latent medical problem, but his primary purpose in such an encounter is to serve as a social gatekeeper. When the physician faces a patient with venereal disease, the patient must be treated, but the physician is obligated to look beyond the patient and show concern for the social order as well. The physician whose patient has a new, un-studied problem necessarily is torn between his devotion to that particular patient and obligations to the body of professional knowledge which may help many other patients. Does the physician intervene immediately or sit watchfully as the problem plays out its "natural course"? Contracting economies encourage some to run up the banner of "cost containment" which "will force the physician to make painful choices between individual care and stewardship of the limited resources of society."[2] Technical advances such as the ability to assess fetal genetic make-up early in a pregnancy force physicians to face the question, "For whom do I work? The fetus or the family? The family or the society which will have to subsidize care of a defective child?"

The answers to such questions are not clear, but medicine is casting about for satisfactory solutions to the dilemma posed by conflicting obligations in the medical encounter. Some physicians want to design a health care system in which they can be technicians and can leave the economic, political, social and psychological aspects of care to others. So, for example, Robert Murray encouraged his colleagues to support extra-medical "screening and counseling programs where individual rights and values are given first priority."[3] He envisioned a division of labor in which the physician would be simply a technician who leaves decisions about who should get what care to others. Murray and Burnam respond in one voice when placed in the position of being a double agent: they will "leave it to a separate advocate of the state to rank [their] patients according to their worthiness to receive care."[4]

The isolationist perspective of Murray and Burnam has gained little support in medicine since doctors feel obligated, and most appear willing, to face the challenges of their own logic, which forces them to look in two directions at once. Instead of resolving its dilemma by dissolving one of the dilemma's poles, medicine has attempted to formulate an internal solution in which actions responsive to the demands of the social order do not appear to contravene the physician's obligations to the patient.

To resolve the problem of double agentry created by medicine's new logic, the profession has opened a search for models for order that might allow physicians to rationalize difficult individual decisions in terms of the larger order. At this stage, three lines of inquiry that point toward a vision of order are open and are, to different degrees, being incorporated into medical discourse. Ethics proposes one route to harmony and has held a prominent place in medical discourse for more than a decade. Sociobiology offers another approach to formulating a model for order. Medicine recognizes this new field's potential but only flirts with its language and ideas. The sociobiological form of argument appears in some areas of medical inquiry, but the marriage of disciplines is not yet made. Finally, there is renewed interest in spirituality in and around things medical. Spirituality as an approach to the problem of order sits at the edge of the medical encounter waiting for an opening to appear.

The ethics of care became problematic and began to get a lot of play in the medical press around 1970. That is not to say that medicine was unconcerned with medical ethics before 1970, but it means that discussions of ethical issues changed character around that time.

Modern medicine recognized the importance of professional ethics from its earliest days. Codes of ethics served as organizational devices and checks on the behavior of physicians who otherwise found themselves in destructive competition with one another. So, for example, the Code of Ethics adopted by the fledgling American Medical Association in 1847 specified when physicians should divulge information about patients to other institutions, on what basis physicians were to charge for services, and to whom physicians could and could not refer patients for specialized care (and how fees were to be set when a patient was referred elsewhere). The ethical concerns of medicine during its first century or so were internal concerns, and the profession conducted discussions of ethical issues internally. Questions of how physicians ought to behave toward one another and toward the rest of society were paramount, but they were questions only physicians could (or would be allowed to) answer.

The AMA revised its Principles of Ethics several times. In 1949

the Principles looked outward to an environment beginning to en-
croach on professional discretion with federal regulations and third
party payer schemes. The 1949 Principles was an assertion that no
laws should be made "which would violate professional ethics and
which would incidentally put the independent practitioner at a competitive disadvantage."[5] Then in 1957 the AMA adopted a parallel
Principles, a code that did not replace the 1949 but sat alongside
it, aimed toward the public. Jeffrey Berlant, a physician who took
a Ph.D. in sociology, argues that the 1949 and 1957 codes demonstrate that the social use of ethical codes has changed from a
"means for ordering the conduct of physicians to a means for
legitimizing the monopolistic privileges of the profession to the
powers-that-be and to the public."[6] This change in orientation is
but one side of the changes in the character of ethical discourse in
medicine.

When it shifted its audience, around 1950, from fellow professionals to those on whom maintenance of professional privilege
rested, medical ethics was exposed to the contentiousness of the
environment in which medicine operates. Discussion of medical-
ethical issues began to churn during the 1950s and erupted in 1970.
Suddenly the character of care was open for discussion, and nonmedical personnel, particularly ethicists, became party to that
discussion.

It was in 1970 that Daniel Callahan and his colleagues founded
the Institute of Society, Ethics, and Life Sciences. Braving the
hostility of some sectors of the profession of medicine and the
cross-disciplinary wariness of one another, people from many fields
joined together to form an Institute to examine new ethical problems in a "sober, systematic and professional way."[7]

It was also around 1970 that medical journals began publishing
physicians' discussions of ethically problematic practices within
the hitherto sacrosanct doctor-patient dyad. For example, in 1973
the *New England Journal* published two controversial papers on
ethical dilemmas in the treatment of children. Raymond Duff and
A. G. M. Campbell[8] documented the extent of deaths from pur-

posefully discontinued care in neonatal intensive care nurseries, while Anthony Shaw outlined ethical problems that arise in treating the young, illustrating his points with a number of cases taken from his own practice.[9] These papers were but a part of the explosion in the discussion of ethical problems that occurred little more than a decade ago.

What was the fuss about? Callahan's interdisciplinary group "thought that acrimonious ethical disagreement, on the one hand, and uncertainty about ethical goals on the other, were . . . beginning to pose obstacles to the future development of medicine. . . . Questions of ethics and values, if left unattended, have a way of festering when, as is often the case, they are not examined and treated."[10] Most people claim that the acrimonious debate and festering sores of modern medicine arose from technological developments that allowed the profession to detect medical problems earlier, refine prognoses, and sustain "life" longer than ever before. This "technological determinism" is a weak argument. Technological developments create ethical problems only in the context of a medical logic that makes the doctor's obligations ambiguous and open to questions from others. A monastic medicine would face exactly the same situations as modern medicine faces, but it would not face the same ethical problems. Dissension might arise internally, but it was in the nature of monastic medicine to contain dissension and resolve differences without allowing scrutiny from the outside.

The traditional physician, locked in the traditional fiduciary doctor-patient relationship operating under the rule of silence, faces an unproblematic situation as he stands over a hyper-instrumented patient who is consuming enormous amounts of medical resources. The doctor's obligations to the patient are clear and unquestionable. In contrast, the modern physician who must be simultaneously responsive to the patient and responsible for the social order is overwhelmed with problems—ethical problems—in the same situation. His obligations are not clear. Should therapy be discontinued if the family's financial resources will suffer irreparable damage? Should life be sustained when the excruciatingly painful disruptions in the social circle around the patient become evident? What does a doctor say to a pregnant woman carrying a fetus with Down's Syndrome when the woman refuses to have an abortion if the chances that the child will be institutionalized for life, at society's expense, are, say, 50–50? Technological advances create these situations; the logic of medicine makes the obligations of the physician ambiguous, and the ambiguity, in turn, makes the situation ethically problematic.

As if the problem of being made a double agent were not enough, a profession accorded by its logic responsibility for social order will inevitably find itself in conflict with other professions and social institutions which presume to have the same responsibility. Callahan said, "If ethical issues were left unattended and unexamined, one would have to expect public suspicion, ill informed legislative incursions, and emotional clashes within and outside of the profession."[11] There would be no reason to expect less. A legislature with a constitutional mandate to preserve order would resent the incursion of medicine into its domain and could reasonably be expected to respond in kind. A republic founded on democratic rhetoric could reasonably be expected to respond at least with suspicion to a privileged monopoly that presumed to answer fundamental questions of right action in matters of life, death, family dynamics, economic well-being, and social order. Medicine's own logic has thrown medicine into conflict with other venerable institutions, placed its practices on view and opened the profession up for examination.

The cost to modern medicine of accepting the mantle of an expanded calling has been the disharmony that inevitably results when an institution, whose stability depended on the existence of a mandate with clear limits, oversteps its boundary. The disharmony we now see around modern medicine is not unlike the disharmony caused by Monte Lupo's priest throwing open the doors of the church and marching through the town for which he felt responsible and for which he wanted to do something besides pray earnestly but quietly behind the church walls. Once the priest steps out of his church or the doctor steps out of the clinic, disharmony results.

Enter ethics.

Discussion of ethical issues in medical care seeks to harmonize a situation fraught with disharmony. Stephen Toulmin, an ethicist writing in 1950, said, "what makes us call a judgment 'ethical' is the fact that it is used to harmonize people's actions."[12] Twenty-five years later another ethicist echoed these sentiments exactly when he pointed out to medicine, "the object of ethics is a harmonious and just society."[13] And the sociologist Talcott Parsons felt no hesitation in drawing the following equivalence, "I shall treat the question of ethics as essentially one of social responsibility—that is, responsibility to promote or at least do no harm to the values and welfare of the social system and the various classes of its members."[14] The holon that represents medicine's expanded scope of attention but which also embodies the ambiguities of medicine's calling is ordered. Through discussion of ethically difficult situations one hopes to arrive at ethically acceptable courses of action that respect and maintain the order of the holon while the physician discharges his or her duties to the patient.

Ethics does not propose, however, to trample over the individualism medical logic so carefully created. In fact, if the support group is the social form that mediates between the individual and the social order, it is the action of ethical systems that keeps individualism from dissolving in a social order and the social order from degenerating into anarchic individualism. Ethics complements the support group by keeping separate that which the support group would link together, the individual and the social order.

Writing about physicians who engaged certain patients—people burned so badly that survival was unprecedented—in decisions about their care, Eric Cassell severed connection with traditional medicine when he said, "the job of medicine is not merely to save life but rather is the preservation of autonomy."[15] Autonomy is achieved, as in the support group, by fostering a sense of control in the patient by forming an effective patient-physician partnership. Cassell said, "physicians do not sustain hope promising the cure of disease or survival (which patients often know is not possible). Rather, they sustain hope by keeping patients as much in command of themselves, their symptoms and their situation as possible." But, paradoxically, this independence derives from a partnership: "autonomy for the sick patient cannot exist outside of a good and properly functioning doctor-patient relation. And the relation between them is inherently a partnership."[16] An ethical solution to the problem of order thrusts the patient's individuality in his or her face and "lets" him or her make those difficult decisions which will preserve order even if the price to be paid is the patient's own death. Ethics contributes to those disciplinary mechanisms that cause one to become true to his own nature. It is only reasonable, the argument would go, that a person burned to the point where survival is unprecedented should choose to die. Death is in the nature of people whose survival is unprecedented.

One might object to the seeming rigidity of this characterization of the new medical decision-making process that involves the patient. One might object to the assumption that the patient will necessarily make decisions about care that respect social order. But in the new therapeutic alliance, in the inherent partnership of patient and physician, what else is the patient to decide? To answer that rhetorical question we must add the crucial caveat to descriptions of the new physician, the new patient, and the new doctor-patient relationship developed to this point. The physician must, according to medicine's new logic, recognize and respect the individuality of the patient, and the new patient does enter into a joint adventure with the physician; but, as we said earlier, patient and physician alike are subordinated to a higher vision of order. The physician may be a person who negotiates care[17] with another person, the patient; but negotiations in the new therapeutic alliance must proceed with the intention of discovering together the true order of the holon. The ethically responsible physician will foster an individual's autonomy by joining in partnership as long as the individual enters into that partnership reasonably (i.e., with reason), for it is only through reason that true order can be discovered.

The patient interview, discussed above, is not simply structured like a confessional; patient and physician are compelled to act out a confession. The patient must enter the interview in the same way the penitent enters the Christian confessional. The task of the interview is not to celebrate the individual with his or her peculiar problems; the task is to extract a patient's individuality, locate the patient in terms of deviations from optimal life courses, and seek strategies for normalizing those deviations so that the patient can achieve a true and fulfilling life course trajectory. Modern medical logic no longer claims to know life through the act of seeing, which it first enunciated by adopting the anatomy lesson as its logo. Nevertheless, life still has a knowable shape, form and definition. It has empirical limits that define it. Beyond those limits, speech fails and falls into the sometimes confusing, sometimes perilous, and always wrong domain of unreason. Thus, medicine in the new mold shares with traditional medicine an intolerance for the unreal and unreasonable: the patient who unreasonably demands to be kept alive when there is no hope of survival, the parents who can't really want a defective child to be born. These exist beyond the limits of life tamed by reason, and these cannot be tolerated. The physician and patient who enter into a therapeutic alliance are thereby pledged to reason together to find the ethically appropriate, socially harmonious course of action.

Finding an ethically appropriate course of action does not require either doctor or patient to be superhuman as the professionalization of "medical ethics" might lead one to believe. Despite myriad ethical theories and the insistence of ethicists that ethics is not simply a matter of one person's opinion versus another's opinion and that "there are better ways and worse ways to accomplish [the] harmonizing task,"[18] those same ethicists tell us that there is nothing special or privileged or difficult about ethical reasoning. Clouser says, "We [ethicists] are not calling on some special sense of morality, but only on the principles or moral rules that we ordinarily acknowledge in everyday life." Ethicists, he says, can merely help "structure" issues: " 'Structuring' the issues is an analytical dissection. It is a road map of the issue, showing routes, relations, functions, shortcuts, and central and peripheral locations. It shows you where various arguments and actions lead, what facts would be relevant, what concepts are crucial, and what moral principles are at issue and probably in conflict."[19] Ethicists simply try to elaborate the true nature of a situation, its rich morphological contours and its finest details, so that no deceit, no personal interests, and no extraneous issues of any sort can interfere with the force of reason as action is decided. But, ethicists tell us, anyone willing to reason well and think dispassionately can accomplish the same end.

Whereas the eyes were critical to traditional medicine since the eyes made death and disease visible and directed the informed gaze to its targets in the body, their importance is diminished under a logic which demands that invisible relationships between the body and all other things be made available for evaluation and medical work. Disciplined reason, not well instructed eyes, is the basis of the new informed "gaze." Reason makes invisible relationships visible and directs action toward them. One physician who argued that only parents, siblings, physicians and nurses should be considered in the care of a radically defective infant, and that the interests of the infant itself should not enter into medical decisions at all, said, "The child itself . . . is not a person, and the fundamental error of our ways consists in thinking that it is one. The problem underlying our natural error is that *we trust what we see and not what we know.*"[20] Reason, he argued, should override the senses, for it is only reason, not the senses, that has access to the relationships and invisible structures toward which medical decisions are now directed.

The discipline of ethics claims it can help elaborate the structure of difficult issues by making invisible relationships visible. It seeks a limited partnership with medicine for the purpose of improving ethical decision making in medical care, but discussion of ethical issues in medicine has recently taken a curious turn. Consider, for example, the conclusion of a bold and controversial paper on "Indicators of Humanhood" in which noted ethicist Joseph Fletcher sets out his list of criteria for according something the status "human." After listing specific (a minimum score of 20 on a standard I.Q. test), general (a "balance of rationality and feeling"), positive (capable of relating to others), and negative (not essentially parental or sexual) criteria for acquiring humanness in the eyes of others, he concludes by saying: "I rather suspect we are more apt to find good answers inductively and empirically, from medical science and the clinicians, than by the necessarily syllogistic reasoning of the humanities. . . . Divorced from the laboratory and the hospital, talk about what it means to be human could easily become inhumane."[21] Fletcher is appealing to reason of a special sort—the reason of science, the laboratory, and, in particular, the reason of biology. It is as if the order of the holon were a natural order whose truth can be apprehended by seeing deeply—much more deeply than Vesalius, Morgagni, Leeuwenhoek, or the Curies ever conceived of seeing—into our biological selves. Fletcher is suggesting that if we can see very deeply into the biochemical basis of life, we will probably apprehend there the laws of a natural order for the holon. And if we follow this line of thinking carefully, we soon confront the rhetorical question, what law could be more compelling than a law whose base is not social consensus or the power of a prince but rather the biological foundation of what we are?

Why the language, methods, and conclusions of the new discipline of sociobiology are seeping into medical discourse is now clear. Sociobiology extends the Darwinian argument based on mutation and natural selection to include notions of ecological interaction—the setting and processes in which natural selection takes place—and production—which links the genotype or genetic constitution of an organism with its phenotype, its appearance.[22] A logic based in these two concepts extends the medical gaze from the disease located in the body, which has a history reconstructable in terms of mechanical and chemical events, to the social order.

The social order consists of unique phenotypic individuals "produced" by their unique genotypic constitutions, which have a history reconstructable in terms of interactions in an ecology over long periods of time. Naturally, the language of sociobiology would appeal to a medicine whose logic has forced it to expand its scope of attention but whose history has left it without a language for dealing with all that now falls within its purview but with a tradition steeped in a language of events produced by essential forces and structures.

E. O. Wilson's *Sociobiology: The New Synthesis,* published in 1975, reinvigorated the discipline that had lain dormant since the last part of the nineteenth century.[23] Sociobiology, according to Wilson, "is defined as the systematic study of the biological basis of all forms of social behavior, including sexual and parental, in all kinds of organisms, including humans."[24] Wilson's large book differed from those of his nineteenth century counterparts in the degree of sophistication he could bring to the study of social behavior, but, more important, it differed in the amount of space it devoted to the study of humans. Wilson bracketed a massive, scholarly accumulation of knowledge of animal behavior with two short chapters on human behavior. Nineteenth century sociobiologists, had they had that term to call themselves, would have been appalled by Wilson's apparent timidity and reserve in making connections between animal behavior and human behavior that, to them, would have been self-evident. In contrast, Wilson's twentieth century critics were appalled that he would so boldly march into human behavior and be so brash as to make the kinds of statements, however limited, he did about humans.

What did Wilson do to so offend the sensibilities of so many social scientists, biologists, and other contemporary students of social behavior? Put simply, Wilson tried to suggest that our social order has its basis in biology. Wilson's last chapter, "The Morality of the Gene," initiated a search for the biological base for morality and ethics, the glue that keeps a rather fragile social order from falling apart. "There is an underlying unity of human experience,"[25] sociobiology tells us, and it is the task of the sociobiologist to cut through the vast, obvious cultural diversity we observe in the world to discover the truth all humans share in the depths of their biological selves. "The sociobiologist is interested in the more general features of human nature and the limitations that exist in the environmentally induced variations. He or she is especially interested in the fact that, although all cultures taken together constitute a very great amount of variation, their total content is far less than that displayed by the remaining species of social animals."[26] The underlying unity—the unity displayed in human social behavior to the informed gaze of the sociobiologist—once isolated, must be biologically based. This, at least, is the argument of sociobiology.

Sociobiology extends Darwin's idea that individual traits have a biological base and evolve through natural selection to say that social traits, particularly social traits that effect order, have a biological base and evolve through ecological interaction. For example, Lionel Tiger believes that the root of order is optimism and speaks of optimism as an essential part of human nature: "making optimistic symbols and anticipating optimistic outcomes in undecided situations is as much part of human nature, of the human biology, as are the shape of the body, the growth of children, and the zest of sexual pleasure."[27] Optimism is something that gets passed on, like eye color, through natural selection in an active ecology: "Optimists were [in past millennia] more likely to cope and reproduce than pessimists, other things being equal; an important root of social cohesion and economic innovation is as biologically understandable as the sweating that accompanies fear, though far less tangible and immediate."[28] George Pugh, whose work on values was written contemporaneously with Wilson's *Sociobiology,* says that sociobiological theory "suggests that our fundamental human values are not an accident or a mystery but rather a natural and almost inevitable consequence of evolution's basic 'design concept' for the brain." Like Wilson, Pugh believes that altruism is the basis for social order and that altruism is, like optimism and eye color, passed on: "The new perspectives seem generally to support the altruistic principles of Western religion and modern humanism. Indeed, many of our traditional social values such as 'freedom,' 'justice,' 'equity,' and the concept of 'right and wrong' seem to follow as almost automatic consequences of theory."[29]

Sociobiology suggests that social and personal values, both innate, interact over time, and as a result of this interaction social ethical systems "evolve" to mediate between the individual and the social order. "Wilson specifically considers ethics as a branch of evolutionary biology; our cherished human values are to be judged in terms of their effect on the survival of the genes of those individuals who live according to our ethical precepts. . . ."[30] It is the step from explaining human behavior to proposing guidance for human actions by elevating the biological component of ethical behavior above the social component that bothers so many critics of sociobiology,[31] but it is precisely this elevation of the biological that makes sociobiological reasoning attractive to medicine and allows medicine to leech off sociobiology as it searches for models for order.

Sociobiological reasoning contains both tracks of medical logic— the individual and the social order—and resolves any ambiguous or conflicting commitments to one or the other by understanding both in neo-Darwinian, evolutionary terms. First, there is an emphasis on the absolute uniqueness of the individual. Speaking at a conference on the biological basis of criminality, Henry E. Kelly said that a biochemical approach to crime prevention could start with "the concept of biochemical individuality. This concept states that we humans . . . though similar in our biological and biochemical composition, are absolutely unique."[32] Once again, this is not said to celebrate the individual. Instead, it is said to make more acceptable the normalizing, biochemical interventions into human behavior that are constructed to insure social order and social stability. "It may be that as the biological causes [of crime and disorder] are found and treated [virtually] all citizens would see the goals and means and rewards and punishments provided by advanced capitalist societies to be sufficient for them to conform. Thus, the problem may not be the coming large-scale biochemical control of a population, but the discovery that it is only needed on a very small scale—and under the legitimation of health and happiness and respectability by natural means."[33] What could be more appealing to modern medicine than a discipline which recognizes the individual above all else but then, in the name of health and happiness, intervenes in small, simple, natural, and highly individualized ways to insure that the individual fits well into the order around him?

Some critics have attacked sociobiology for equating the social order we have "evolved"—the order of "advanced capitalist societies" to use Kelly's phrase—with a morally imperative "good" to be defended by any means necessary. This is an inappropriate criticism of the discipline, for sociobiologists, being schooled in the limitations as well as the advantages of scientific reasoning, generally do not make the leap from scientific explanation to moral imperative. Their message is more subtle, more morally benign, but they do not intend their message to be any less compelling for it. Sociobiology argues simply that if we, as free and willful yet social beings, try to construct social orders different from the one that has evolved around us, we will face, first, difficulty and, second, disastrous consequences. Wilson says that human behavior is narrowly constrained if compared to the wide variation found in forms of social behavior among animals, and he recognizes that we could, in principle, change our forms of human organization using animal behavior as a model if we wished. But he cautions, "Even if we were to attempt to duplicate some of these [animal] social behaviors by conscious design, it would be a charade likely to create emotional breakdown and a rapid reversal of effort."[34] Life must align itself with the norms that define it. People must become true to their own natures.

Respect for community and social order as we find it are keys to realizing individuality and happiness in the modern world, according to sociobiology. Kai Erikson, a sociologist but not a sociobiologist, wrote after studying the social effects of a flood, "It is the community that cushions pain, the community that provides a context for intimacy, the community that represents morality."[35] Sociobiology does not tell us to respect the order-inducing, community-oriented potentialities in our genes because, in liturgical rhetoric, "it is good that we do so," but because if we do not do so we will lose the very cornerstone of our existence as individuals, the social order. The language and reasoning of sociobiology resolves the dilemma created by the new medical logic by making individualism and uniqueness dependent on the individual having a well integrated place in the social order and by locating the laws of that social order in the genetic endowment of the individual. Life becomes identical to maps of relationships between subsystems and suprasystems and is created as something suspended in these web-like maps.

Sociobiology does not suggest that human beings are unwillful or unpurposeful. People have desires that go well beyond basic biological needs, some of which are easily realized, others of which exist as more or less engaging visions. Sociobiology, though, conceives of a world "in which each person will have only desires that are compatible with the satisfaction of the desires of others."[36] This was the vision of nineteenth century sociologists and it remains the vision that informs sociobiology today. The difference is that nineteenth century intellectuals located the compelling forces that were to regulate disorderly desires—that is, the passions which have no patience for the desires of others—in social laws, while in the twentieth century we seem to wish to locate the laws on which order depends in biology.

Medicine is only beginning to incorporate the language and reasoning of sociobiology into medical discourse. Physicians are beginning to tell one another, "the gene has implications not only for all aspects of the science of humankind but also for the social, political, and cultural aspects of human activity." The transmission of genetic information is cited as the model for the transmission of information and communication in the medical encounter. And they say, "human behavior is probably as finely ordered as organic molecular structure."[37] Medicine has moved somewhat beyond this poetry of order, though, and has started to investigate the (now) medical problems of social disorder relying heavily on sociobiological methods. For example, Marshall Klaus and John Kennell expanded the scope of medicine's interest from the event of "birth" to the post-partum dynamics of "mother-infant interaction." They argued that studies of animals and their own studies of human behavior showed that a woman should desire to behave in specific ways toward her newborn infant so that she and the infant could respect their inherited biogram by becoming "bonded" to one another.[38] Without maternal-infant bonding, physicians and others claimed, all sorts of horrible things could happen including child abuse by unbonded parents, degeneration to a life of crime by the unbonded child, and total disruption of the early year's of the unbonded child's life.[39] Klaus and Kennell later studied the effects of having a supportive companion attend a woman in labor. They claimed that their results showed that, regardless of whether a woman desires to have someone with her during birth, her labor is better from obstetrical and experiential points of view if she does have someone with her.[40] Given data that purport to reveal the truth of our social behavior as it emanates from our biological core, who could possibly choose not to have a supportive companion with her during labor and delivery? Who could desire against scientific truth, especially since it is such reasonable truth? Clearly, only a woman who was unreasonable, that is to say, a woman who cannot accept the force of reason.

Sociobiology offers medicine a mode of access to those invisible relationships existing between bodies to which medicine's attention is directed by its new logic. It provides medicine a vehicle with which to fulfill the obligations of its expanded calling. Whether medicine will fully incorporate sociobiological thinking, data, and conclusions into medical practice remains an empirical question. There is, however, an attractive match between the needs of the new medicine and what sociobiology has to offer.

Sociobiology and medical ethics are two different but slowly converging approaches to the problem of order. To different degrees they are being made part of medical discourse. A third approach to the problem of order is appearing at the edges of medicine and seems to be trying to attract medicine's attention. Briefly stated, a renewed interest in the spiritual dimension of existence is appearing as medicine attempts to discover models for order in secular life.

Not surprisingly, the new language of spirituality appeared first in the death and dying literature. Kenneth Ring, the psychologist whose research on the near-death experience confirmed many of Raymond Moody's claims, sought the meaning of his research results in the spiritual domain. In his scientist's garb Ring sounds very much the sociobiologist. He says, "Most near-death experiences seem to unfold according to a single pattern, almost as though the prospect of death serves to release a stored, common 'program' of feelings, perceptions, and experiences," and, "The definitive physiological and neurological explanation [of near-death experiences] remains to be articulated. Now that the phenomenon itself has been established as a reliable feature of the dying experience, we can only applaud serious scientific research and theorizing in this direction."[41] Then, however, Ring links the scientific and the spiritual, saying, "the modern world of physics and the spiritual world seem to reflect a single reality. If this is true, no scientific account of any phenomenon can be complete without taking its spiritual aspect into account."[42] Following his own claim for the linkage of the scientific and the spiritual, Ring carefully and ostentatiously removes his scientist's smock and offers his own view of the meaning of his data. He says he regards near-death experiences as "teachings," "revelatory experiences." "They vouchsafe both to those who undergo them and to those who hear about them an intuitive sense of the transcendent aspect of their creation. These experiences clearly imply that there is something more, something beyond the physical world of the senses. . . ."[43]

Moody and Kübler-Ross have accompanied Ring this far. They

and others are making appeals for the consideration of spiritual aspects of dying in medical care of dying patients. They insist that modern medicine can only find meaning—or shall we say reason—for its practices by acknowledging the spiritual dimension of living as medicine plys its scientific wares. Psycho-sexual approaches to childbirth are bringing a language of spirituality to the other end of life. The glorious experiences that can be had for the price of sociobiologically surrendering to one's body or of engaging in a few exercises may be cast in secular or sexual terms, but the promise the approach holds out to women takes on an unmistakable spiritual luster.[44]

Insisting that the spiritual dimension be considered in medical care is one way to order a set of systems that constantly faces disorder. The holon hierarchy of systems moves through space and time drawing resources from the environment as necessary and maintaining a fragile equilibrium. Intuitively, death would seem to be the ultimate disruption of the holon. It irreparably shuts down all systems in the body and propagates a new disorder upwards through other systems. To strictly secular modern medicine death represents the ultimate insult and sign of failure; it is the radical break from life for which there is no counteractive, restabilizing intervention in the holon. Introducing spirituality into medical discourse gives the holon another dimension through which it can move. The holon that exists in a world infused with spirituality does not represent "everything" and death does not represent a radical break from life. In a structure where "life" is identical to a normative order or pattern of relationships, death becomes a point of transition, an instantaneous shift from one trajectory to another, a shift from a trajectory through time and space to a trajectory in another dimension "beyond the physical world of the senses" as Ring puts it. Death, once a momentous event, becomes another aspect of the normative structure that is life. The ultimate dislocation caused by death dissolves into a well-ordered scheme constructed in more encompassing terms.

We must not carry this too far. The new practices of medical discourse are being carried out in a mixed language. The incorporation of spirituality, sociobiology and ethics into medical discourse is just beginning, and the history we are living may see a quick reversal of present trends. The future remains an empirical question; we must not constrain it by reading more into this most recent chapter in the history of medicine than the texts permit. Yet the need of modern medicine for a model for order in the face of a new logic that foists conflicting obligations onto the physician is clear. Just as clear is the gathering of different approaches to the problem of order around medicine. Whether medicine will follow the path it has marked out for itself is a question that will only be answered with time.

# Ten

# The Tyranny of Harmony

W E HAVE TRIED to measure the distance between Vesalius's *De Fabrica* and the 1980 edition of *The Principles and Practice of Modern Medicine,* the successor to Sir William Osler's medical text. It was never at issue that between them lay a great accumulation of knowledge, theory and practice. Between Vesalius and the authors of *The Principles and Practice of Modern Medicine* stand an eminent array of great scientists, practitioners, and texts. There is also a broad array of physicians who understood in different ways the power their knowledge and practices gave them over their patients. We have tried to show, however, that only when we understand that *De Fabrica* and *Principles and Practice* represent radically different forms of medical power can we appreciate fully their relation to one another within a particular type of discourse and within the particular institution of medicine.

The type of discourse to which they both belong is one in which life is to be known as a set of structures and functions that have an observable form and unity. It is a discourse that cannot know life in such terms without knowing the empirical form and unity of its nemesis, death, as well. Within the type of discourse to which both *De Fabrica* and *Principles and Practice* belong, medicine gains identity as a set of practices confronting a death that tracks through the body in the form of diseases, something on the order of a wild beast stalking life in order to end it.

What separates *De Fabrica* from *Principles and Practice* are the parameters of that confrontation that each enunciates. *De Fabrica* symbolizes the principles operating almost exclusively until around 1950. Medicine was like a warrior-guardian that stood over life to protect it from death. Death and life belonged to separate dominions connected only by that relationship which connects enemies. Medicine hunted death and made it visible in the world, but simultaneously medicine turned death into a kind of chimerical beast that transfigured itself into a multiplicity of diseases. Medicine applied force mindful of life to contain and circumscribe mindless forces that produced death and tried to protect life from death wherever and whenever possible.

The twentieth edition of *The Principles and Practice of Modern Medicine* represents different principles. Life is no longer to be saved from the wildness of death; the wildness of death is to be tamed in life. Around 1950 the language of modern medicine began to identify the structures of life with the normative order of an ecological system that embraced everything that could be spoken about. Life and death came to occupy the same space. Within that space the wildness of death became something that served as the climax of life. Life was tamed so that it would conform to a normative structure that posits death as its appropriate if not glorious climax. An erotically tinted language that ranged across notions of completion, fulfillment, and joy infused the new medical language that spoke true about life and death.

When all of the components and subsystems and suprasystems of life conform to the order of relationships and information flows that identify the structure of life itself, death is transmogrified and becomes that which does not threaten us but serves us. The image of medicine as a warrior-guardian that protects life from death is transformed into the tamer-trainer of beasts who must watch not only the beast but everything else in the space it occupies. Relationships that were once inconsequential become central. How far am I from the beast? How far is it from the stool? How close are others to each of us? Every tiny detail of the beast's behavior must be monitored, not so its behavior can be changed radically or its movement stopped forcefully but so its behavior can be managed. Only if the entire space—the beast, the trainer, and all else it contains—is properly managed can the beast be taken through the proper sequence of acts that serve the integrity of the larger order and that permit us to apply the designation "tamed." People may still pay to see beasts contained and subdued by force, but today the real money is to be made from proper management that leads one through experientially optimal courses of events that give people a sense of participation in thrilling adventures.

What, though, is tamed? A beast that is well managed is not the same beast that stalks in the wild. That which once threatened life suddenly seems to become bigger than life. Medical logic has caused a great reversal in our thinking, whose archetype is the Frankenstein myth. Death becomes life. We expect to tame life and be happier for it, but the great beast loses none of its fearsomeness. The structures and functions that were divided by death acquire an awesome power to destroy the most cherished aspects of life once they are expertly pieced back together. Life replaces death as the great beast in need of taming, and we will go as far as necessary to hunt it down. In the new logic of medicine, in the new approach of the doctor to the patient, in new conceptions of disease, in medicine's expanded calling and in the emergent concerns for order we can see the profession of medicine adopting the posture of a tamer of life and abandoning the stance of a warrior-guardian pitted against death. And medicine's antagonist now is life, not death.

Over the image of the anatomy lesson a new image has appeared. The new image is not so sharply defined nor as dramatic as the woodcut of Vesalius instructing his audience in the anatomy amphitheater, but we have tried to trace its emerging outlines. A 1980 Mead Johnson and Company advertisement captures many features of this new image (see figure 10.1). What do we see? Instead of an anonymous cadaver we see three vital, clearly individual children. Instead of disease we see problems: protein allergy, feeding prob-

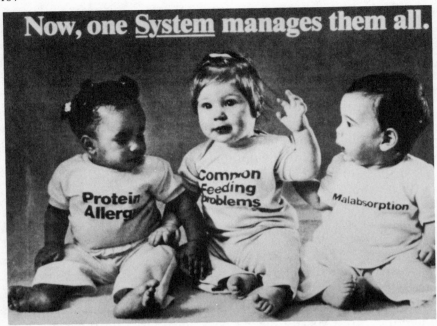

Now, one <u>System</u> manages them all.

FIGURE 10.1 Mead Johnson and Company advertisement, copyright 1980. Reproduced with permission.

lems, and malabsorption problems. Instead of discovering these problems by violently intruding into the spaces of these beautiful bodies, the children announce their problems themselves—typically for our time, on their T-shirts. Instead of treatment and cure we see that the problems are to be managed. And we see that the problems are to be managed by a system developed by a corporate entity.

Where in this image is Vesalius? He is no longer visible. He exists only by inference. His presence can be invoked, but he fades quickly to become a component of the overall management system. He has become like a figure in a pentimento, a ghostly figure that seeps through the dominant form; he is a figure that can be perceived only on closest inspection. This, then, is the new image of medicine painted over the logo of the anatomy lesson. It is not an image that is fully formed yet, nor is it necessarily permanent, but its general features are clear enough.

Medicine has not embraced this new image completely. There is reluctance and occasional hostility to the implications of the eco-logical-systems-theoretic perspective, which recreates patient and physician alike as people and disease as disturbances in integrated but encompassing hierarchies of systems. Everyone, it seems, knows an anecdote about a doctor who, without discussing matters at all, removed a woman's breast or performed a possibly unnecessary hysterectomy, or about a doctor who, in the face of protestations to the contrary, insisted that a patient was doing just fine, right after pulling himself away from computer printouts of laboratory values. Clearly, there is considerable open, organized resistance to alternatives in birth and death even though the opinion leaders of the profession wholeheartedly endorsed some alternatives as early as 1950. The image of Vesalius in his anatomy theater still exists for medicine; the profession is struggling with the ascendant, rather sterile image of the system in which the physician's centrality fades.

Some battles occur after the war is lost, however. Medicine may resist the new dominant image, but it cannot deny the image's compelling force. The obstetrician who today approaches a delivery with the watchful and armed expectancy and the surgico-prophy-lactic techniques of Joseph B. DeLee is nagged by the compulsion of a new image in which the woman is a joint adventurer in an experientially optimal, well managed birth. The physician is not nagged simply because women have combatively thrown this new image in the face of medicine; the physician is nagged because medicine's own logic has thrust the new to the fore. The physician who secludes the dying patient from friends and family behind a screen of Intensive Care Unit rules is nagged by another image of death—not simply because the dying person or the immediate fam-ily insist that dying be handled differently, but because the phy-sician knows that dying can be managed differently and that this would lead to a different death. Medicine can cling to the image of

Vesalius and celebrate the prowess of the anatomist-surgeon, but the profession knows that the image of Vesalius is giving way to the well managed health resource team. The endocrinologist, the immunobiologist, and the genetic counselor are the physicians who will have to be applauded in the coming years.

Medicine can resist its logic, but escaping the new structure of power will be difficult. The walls of monastic medicine within which disease and death could be circumscribed and met with the force of medical reason are gone. Medical practice that operates under the localizing and circumscribing effects of the informed gaze used to be good medicine. The obstetrician who draped women to expose only the obstetrically important parts, who submerged all else under veils of anesthesia, and who transferred interest in the case to the neonatologist immediately after the event used to be doing good work. The spawning of subspecialty upon subspecialty used to be identified with medical progress. No more. An obstetrician must become concerned with postnatal family dynamics. The integrative specialties like family practice, perinatology and immunology are ascendant. Medicine's new calling is more of a compulsion to change its own practice than it is a license to "medicalize" everything.

Whereas the taxonomic approach of medicine constantly narrowed medicine's field of vision, the ecological model and systems-theoretic logic are expanding it. All other parameters of medical practice are changing in response. The health care team extends medicine's reach into many dimensions of life previously closed to medicine. Epidemiology extends medicine's scope of surveillance out into the community. Lay education makes people monitors of their own health and the first line in the detection of many problems. Medicine's tentative yet persistent experiments with alternative means of care—midwife/physician partnerships, hospices, regionalized care programs, community reintegration programs—are broadening the medical umbrella. Even the language of the intensely moral community of monastic medicine is expanding as discourses over the ethics of medical care are incorporated into the hitherto scientifically purified discourse of medical practice.

Medicine's recent history is characterized by a complete reformulation of its field of power. Medicine is not "medicalizing" more aspects of life. That unfortunate term is based on a naive conception of power and implies a form of domination and control that does not adequately capture the nature of medical work today. Nor has medicine ceded some of its power and shared it with other professionals or proponents of "alternative" means of health care only to go around collecting whatever bits and pieces of medical authority remain after "successful challenges" to that authority. That idea, too, rests on a naive conception of power in which those who challenge must either win or lose and in which power is a finite quantity to be gained, held, seized, shared, and generally subjected to the language of zero-sum games. Instead, the field of medical power has changed to become incorporative and rapidly responsive to developments around it. The new field of power is not so much dependent on domination and control as it is on monitoring and surveillance. Finally, the locus of medical power is no longer the hands and eyes of the physician but is instead located in large, pervasive structures that exert their force on physicians and patients alike.

Consider the way in which medicine responds to challenges. Occasionally we see the old exclusionary practices. There remains an apparatus for denoting a drug or procedure as "quackery." However, even at the heart of the machinery that seeks to meet challenges with the power of exclusion we see an ever present "rush to knowledge." The rush to knowledge has replaced the rush to exclude as the principal response to challenges to medicine's authority. Natural childbirth came to the United States just prior to 1950. By 1952, journals were publishing studies of the new approach to birth. The rapidity with which medicine responds to such proposals is striking and is a distinguishing feature of medicine today. Even more striking, if not as entrenched, is the degree of medicine's acceptance of many new ideas and practices. Authorities in some areas are exploring cooperative ventures with independent, lay midwives to insure that women who choose to have home births have recourse to hospital care in case of an obstetrical emergency. The reaction of medicine to the hospice movement can be characterized as benign at worst, supportive at best. Paramedical health team members proliferate. Hospitals hire ethicists to do "applied ethics" in clinical settings. Pain management strategies from psychology—group therapy, biofeedback, conditioning, therapeutic touch—are being incorporated into medicine's repertoire. Thousands of medical studies of traditional healers in our country and other countries have been published since the late 1950s, most of them giving the traditional healer a sympathetic, if somewhat puzzled, treatment. "Holism" has replaced "mechanism" as a central concept in medical discourse. Medicine responds to challenges with a rush to knowledge and then, more often than in the past, moves to incorporate the challenge into orthodox medical practice.

We must be clear about the nature of this incorporative response. Medicine is not simply "coopting" the work of other professionals, nor is it accepting alternative strategems *carte blanche*. Medicine listens to the language of medical paraprofessionals, members of nonmedical professions, and others who present a potential challenge to orthodox medicine; it then filters that language and work through the discursive practices of medicine, translates it through medicine's own rush to knowledge, and makes it politically benign vis-à-vis medicine while simultaneously activating it politically vis-à-vis those who enter the new, expanded medical field of power. So, for example, medicine will accept birthing rooms, but it will tell those who wish to use them why birthing rooms are acceptable and why they should wish to use them, indeed, why women need them. That a woman may anticipate feeling better in a birthing room, that she should desire a comfortable environment in which to go through what she may conceive to be a traumatic event are immaterial considerations. Medicine accepts birthing rooms only if it is able to describe for a woman the birthing room experience and the nature of her desires. "Birthing rooms have been shown to be the best place to give birth," the woman will be told. "Of course, you may be anxious, but 20% of all primiparas married three and one-half years living in a two-bedroom duplex—like you—are, too." Medicine accepts and recites her individual concerns and knows, furthermore, that a few simple exercises, a little relaxation conditioning, and reading a few appropriate books will get her on the proper childbirth track. Medicine is compelled by its own logic to speak *with* the patient and to abandon its arrogant posture of speaking *for* the patient, who must remain silent; both doctor and patient are compelled to speak with one another in a common language around which a field of power forms to govern them both. Beyond the limits of this new field of power there is nothing to be said. By reformulating its field of power to be incorporative, medicine multiplies its paths for the expression of power, makes them finer, more penetrating, and farther reaching.

The efficient operation of a rapidly incorporative field of power depends on technologies of monitoring and surveillance. The rule of silence must be broken in favor of an "incitement to discourse,"[1] as Foucault puts it. For medicine's new field of power to be effective there can be no silence, no hidden recesses allowed to remain invisible and unknown. Once diseases were known as entities in the body that present their own truth to the informed gaze of the physician. He read the signs of disease. Speech only intruded into the search for knowledge under such a structure. Diseases, however, that are disruptions in a complex order do not make themselves immediately known to an informed gaze that need only see them. A dynamic, constantly changing, complex hierarchy of systems must be monitored constantly if significant disruptions are to be noted. The nature of the holon's order must be assessed by extracting its parameters and making them available for analysis. Since speech is the only entree to those parameters, it must be encouraged, or incited. The structure that "respects" the individual is a structure that obligates the individual to declare himself or herself and make visible his or her individual deviations from life course trajectories.

Individuality, according to this logic, consists precisely of the constellation of deviations which locate a person on medicine's large and expanding grid of observations of lives. The woman who awaits the experience of childbirth for which nothing can be considered extraneous has her life wrapped up in that singular process not by choice but by the force of an incorporative medical field of power. Every dark recess of her life must be illuminated by the brilliant light of the new medical logic if she is to benefit from the new, social technologies of normalization—biological, psychological, sociological, spiritual, and so on—available under the medical umbrella.

Medicine does not simply allow patients to speak; medicine requires speech, for only through a patient's declarations are the intimate and private parts of the body as the patient lives it made available for medical praxis. Technologies of domination and control compel silence; technologies of monitoring and surveillance incite discourse. Everything, no matter how trivial it might seem, must be noted, recorded, and made the object of analysis. Less invasive electronic monitoring devices are only the most publicly visible aspects of medicine's new technologies. Epidemiology monitors communities' health while people are made monitors of their own health and illness in day-to-day affairs by lay education. Magazines, television, government-sponsored advertisements, and our social environment instruct everyone in the methods of reason by which significant disruptions in life can be apprehended and reported when necessary.

The new medical field of power is Janus-faced, one side exerting its effects on the patient, the other influencing and regulating the behavior of the physician. Medicine complains that it has never been subject to scrutiny as it is today, and its complaint is justified. With the walls of the monastery down, anyone can look in, examine the work that once used to be contained within, study it and judge it. Technologies of monitoring and surveillance make the intimacies of the patient visible, but they also leave visible records, which make the work of the physician assessable by anyone willing to read the records. Medical power no longer resides in the domination of the informed gaze but is located in the structure of a joint adventure. No longer contained in a Vesalius-like figure and expressed unidirectionally within the confines of the doctor-patient dyad, power is dispersed in a larger structure, but it has become more pervasive, more rapid, and more effective for it.

Governing the structure of power is the image of the good life for which death becomes a climax. Like the parent who asked a counselor to "map out all the schools her [three-year-old] daughter would need to go through in order to graduate from Harvard Law School,"[2] we flock to those people who seem to know—who have been invested with the obligation to know—the path of the good life, and we insist that they map out that life for us. We become objects to ourselves as responsibility for mapping the possibilities of life is passed to another. It goes without saying that the others—the experts—respond positively, if with modest reluctance, to our demands. Medicine, under its mandate of taming the last great beast, has a good start on knowing the nature of the good life. Medical reason maps out normative life courses which propose to convert all momentous, revelatory events into the kind of well managed adventures that Sartre's Roquentin understood are the mark of our time.

Promises of the good life, promises of the good death, and making sense of life and death seem like compelling reasons to accept the call to a joint adventure with medicine. And yet in the modern medical adventure the adventurers always stand at peril of suffering the same fate that one of Graham Greene's protagonists did when "the sense of adventure had leaked away and left only the sense of human pain."[3]

Perhaps we are becoming trapped in an ironic situation. Under the sign of the unacceptability of pain and suffering medicine stands in opposition to disorder. It proposes to decipher the order of the holon (which is no less than everything from quarks to the biosphere), deploy systems of monitoring and surveillance, implement an array of technologies of normalization, and smooth out all disruptions and dislocations in that order. Modern medicine strives for harmony. When a social encounter of any sort is organized under the goal of effecting harmonious living, can the encounter ever end? Endings and beginnings become unthinkable. But, then, is it not the endings and beginnings of living things and not deviations from normative trajectories that demarcate their individuality? Can humans know their individuality without beginning to hear themselves speak for themselves while knowing at the same time that what they have begun must with certainty come to an end?

Perhaps it is time to consider the possibility that we must live, as Alfred North Whitehead observed, "with superficial orderings from diverse arbitrary starting points."[4] Perhaps an institution that proposes to install harmony in the place of confrontation, threat, and the other faces of potential disorder is proposing, simply, a "tyranny of harmony."[5] The other side of a tyranny of harmony, we are told, is a free and humane society, "the true measure [of which] is not so much the extent to which harmony and virtue prevail in it as the degree to which its members have a disciplined capacity to live with the jangling evil that is the underside of its freedom, but without ever ceasing to oppose it."[6] We wonder if one need love death in order to come to terms with it or whether coming to terms with death need be defined solely as taming life to serve us. What it would mean for medicine to act in accord with the requisites of a "free and humane society" rather than a harmonious one, not wishing to defeat disease and death but struggling to live with them, is not clear, but it seems a question worth considering.

# Notes

CHAPTER ONE

1. Rodney M. Coe, *Sociology of Medicine,* 2d ed., New York: McGraw-Hill, 1978, p. 3.

2. William R. Rosengren, *Sociology of Medicine: Diversity, Conflict, and Change,* New York: Harper and Row, 1980, p. 4.

3. Thomas S. Szasz and Marc H. Hollander, "A Contribution to the Philosophy of Medicine: The Basic Models of the Doctor-Patient Relationship," *Archives of Internal Medicine* 97 (1956): 585–592.

4. Michel Foucault, "The Subject and Power," *Critical Inquiry* 8 (1982): 777–795, p. 777.

5. Ibid.

6. Ibid., p. 778.

7. Edward W. Said, *Beginnings: Intention and Method,* New York: Basic Books, 1975, p. 288.

8. Byron J. Good and Mary-Jo DelVecchio-Good, "The Semantics of Medical Discourse," pp. 177–212 in E. Mendelson and Y. Elkana, eds., *Sciences and Cultures: Sociology of the Sciences,* Volume 5, Boston: D. Reidel, 1981, p. 181.

9. Peter L. Berger and Thomas Luckmann, *The Social Construction of Reality,* New York: Anchor Books, 1967; Erving Goffman, *Encounters,* Indianapolis, Ind.: Bobbs-Merrill, 1961.

10. Michel Foucault, "Two Lectures," pp. 78–108 in Colin Gordon, ed., *Power/Knowledge: Selected Interviews and Other Writings, 1972–1977,* New York: Pantheon, 1980, p. 89.

11. Michel Foucault, *Discipline and Punish: The Birth of the Prison,* London: Allen Lane, 1977, p. 194.

12. Michel Foucault, *The History of Sexuality, Volume 1—An Introduction,* New York: Pantheon, 1978, pp. 7–8.

CHAPTER TWO

1. Hoyle Leigh and Morton F. Reiser, *The Patient: Biological, Psychological, and Social Dimensions of Medical Practice,* New York: Plenum, 1980, p. vii.

2. Rodney M. Coe, *Sociology of Medicine,* 2d ed., New York: McGraw-Hill, 1978, p. 8.

3. Bernard Barber, "Compassion in Medicine: Toward New Definitions and New Institutions," *New England Journal of Medicine* 295 (1976): 939–943, p. 939.

4. Michel Foucault, *The Birth of the Clinic: An Archeology of Medical Perception,* New York: Pantheon, 1973, p. xii.

5. Stanley Joel Reiser, *Medicine and the Reign of Technology,* Cambridge: Cambridge University Press, 1978, p. 1.

6. Ibid.

7. Ibid., p. 18.

8. Ibid., p. 19.

9. Alice Stewart Trillin, "Of Dragons and Garden Peas: A Cancer Patient Talks to Doctors," *New England Journal of Medicine* 30 (1981): pp. 699–700.

10. Ludwig Choulant, *History and Bibliography of Anatomic Illustration,* Chicago, Ill.: University of Chicago Press, 1920, p. 178.

11. L. R. Lind, trans., *The Epitome of Andreas Vesalius,* New York: Macmillan, 1949, p. xx.

12. Reiser, 1978, p. 15.

13. Quoted in Jacob Needleman, *A Sense of the Cosmos,* New York: Doubleday, 1975, p. 38.

14. John Farquhar Fulton, *Logan Clendening Lectures on the History and Philosophy of Medicine,* Lawrence, Kansas: University of Kansas Press, 1950, p. 18.

15. Reiser, 1978, p. 11.

16. Georges Canguilhem, *On the Normal and the Pathological,* Boston: D. Reidel, 1978, pp. 46–47.

17. René Leriche, 1936, quoted in ibid., p. 46.

18. Plate 2.1 is a photograph of the original frontispiece from *De Fabrica* published in 1543. It and the other woodcuts in *De Fabrica* are by Jean de Calcar, a pupil of Titian. Plate 2.2 is a photograph of the frontispiece of the 1653 edition of the same work. The differences between the later edition and the earlier one are striking. The later version is artistically inferior to the early version. There is much less attention to detail and much less concern for the effects of light. In the early version the bowels of the cadaver are clear, detailed, almost grotesque. Their effect in the later edition has been muted. The skeleton becomes much more important as it carries a scythe instead of a staff and it no longer points out death in the abdomen but points away from the corpse. Vesalius also becomes much more important. His head is disproportionately large in the 1653 edition and he is more obviously engaged in instruction. The tendency of the later picture is to direct attention away from the dead star and toward the picture's constituent elements. Perhaps the most glaring difference, though, is the change in the nude figure clinging in terror to the column in the upper left in 1543. By 1653 he is clothed and indifferent to the spectacle before him. In sum, the seventeenth century version of the anatomy lesson is a more conservative scene than its sixteenth century counterpart.

19. Ernst A. Cassirer, "The Place of Vesalius in the Culture of the Renaissance," pp. 9–20 in *The Four Hundredth Anniversary Celebration of the De Humani Corporis Fabrica of Andreas Vesalius,* The Historical Library, Yale University School of Medicine, 1943, p. 14.

20. See William Ray Arney, *Power and the Profession of Obstetrics,* Chicago, Ill.: University of Chicago Press, 1982.

21. Dr. Charles B. Coventry, Professor of Obstetrics at Geneva College in New York, is reported to have said in 1850 that he "conceives of no purpose, that has for its object the saving of human life, [that] can be either indecorous or immoral." (Frederick T. Parsons, stenographer, *Report of the Trial: The People versus Dr. Horatio N. Loomis for Libel,* Buffalo, N.Y.: Jewitt, Thomas and Co., 1850, p. 26.)

22. Cassirer, 1943, p. 15.

23. Paul Klemperer, "Introduction" to *Seats and Causes of Disease Investigated by Anatomy, In Five Books, Translated from the Latin of John Baptist Morgagni,* New York Academy of Medicine, New York: Hafner Publishing Company, 1960, p. vii.

24. Ivan Illich, *Medical Nemesis: The Expropriation of Health,* New York: Pantheon, 1976, p. 177.

25. Reiser, 1978, p. 91.

26. Ibid., p. 17.

27. Foucault, 1973, p. 142.

28. Ibid., p. 144.

29. Reiser, 1978, p. 91.

30. Canguilhem, 1978, p. 151.

31. Ibid., p. 13.

32. Foucault, 1973, p. 119.

33. Quoted in Qwesi Temkin, "Basic Science, Medicine and the Romantic Era," *Bulletin of the History of Medicine* 37 (1963): 97–130, p. 106.

34. Foucault, 1973, p. 130.

35. Ibid., p. 136.

36. Canguilhem, 1978, p. 12.

37. Ibid.

38. Ibid.

39. Arney, 1982, p. 23.

40. Ibid., p. 24.

41. Ibid., p. 23.

42. Ibid., p. 24.

43. Ibid.

44. Ibid., p. 70.

45. Ibid., p. 71.

46. Michel Foucault, "Introduction" to Canguilhem, 1978, p. xix.

47. Quoted in Needleman, 1975, pp. 14–15.

48. Needleman, 1975, p. 44.

49. Canguilhem, 1978, pp. 12–13.

50. Ibid., p. 13.

51. Foucault, 1978, p. xiv.

52. Susan Sontag, *Illness as Metaphor,* New York: Farrar, Strauss, and Giroux, 1977, p. 66.

53. Foucault, 1973, p. 146.

54. Ibid., p. xviii.

55. Ibid., p. xii.

56. Ibid., p. x.

57. Anton Pavlovich Chekhov, "Ward No. 6," reprinted in abridged

form in Thomas S. Szasz, ed., *The Age of Madness: The History of Involuntary Hospitalization Presented in Selected Texts,* Garden City, N.Y.: Anchor Books, 1973.

58. Foucault, 1973, p. xiv.

CHAPTER THREE

1. Michael Balint, *The Doctor, His Patient and the Illness,* New York: International Universities Press, 1957, p. 216.

2. Barrie R. Cassileth, Robert V. Zupkis, Katherine Sutton-Smith, and Vicki March, "Information and Participation Preferences among Cancer Patients," *Annals of Internal Medicine* 92 (1980): 832–836, p. 832.

3. Philippe Ariès, *The Hour of Our Death,* New York: Vintage Books, 1982, p. 564.

4. Ibid., p. 565.

5. Ibid., p. 566.

6. Ibid.

7. Ibid., p. 567.

8. Robert Blauner, "The Organization of Death," pp. 544–547 in Howard D. Schwartz and Cary S. Kart, eds., *Dominant Issues in Medical Sociology,* Reading, Mass.: Addison-Wesley, 1978.

9. Philippe Ariès, *Western Attitudes toward Death,* Baltimore, Md.: Johns Hopkins University Press, 1974, p. 14.

10. Ivan Illich, *Medical Nemesis: The Expropriation of Health,* New York: Pantheon, 1976, p. 195.

11. Ariès, 1982, pp. 8–9.

12. Ibid., p. 11.

13. Ariès, 1974, p. 25.

14. Ibid., p. 28.

15. Illich, 1976, p. 176.

16. Ariès, 1974, p. 27.

17. Ibid., pp. 45–46.

18. Illich, 1976, p. 177.

19. Ibid., p. 180.

20. Ibid., p. 181.

21. Ariès, 1982, p. 18.

22. Ibid., p. 8.

23. Ibid.

24. Ibid., p. 18.

25. Ibid., p. 16.

26. Ibid., p. 95.

27. Ibid.

28. Ibid., p. 606.

29. Ibid., p. 604.

30. Ibid., p. 370.

31. Ibid., p. 373.

32. Ibid., p. 446.

33. Ariès, 1974, p. 12.

34. Ibid., p. 12.

35. Ibid., p. 11.

36. Ibid., pp. 51–52.

37. Ariès, 1982, p. 107.

38. Ibid., p. 108.

39. Ibid., p. 109.

40. Illich, 1976, p. 184.

41. Ibid., p. 186.

42. Carlos Castaneda, *Journey to Ixtlan: The Lessons of Don Juan,* New York: Pocket Books, 1972, pp. 26–36.

43. Lyn H. Lofland, *The Craft of Dying: The Modern Face of Death,* Berkeley, Calif.: Sage, 1978, p. 17.

44. Ariès, 1974, pp. 4–5.

45. Ariès, 1982, p. 561.

46. Erwin H. Ackerknecht, "Death in the History of Medicine," *Bulletin of the History of Medicine* 42 (1968): 19–24, p. 19.

47. Ariès, 1982, pp. 568–570.

48. Ackerknecht, 1968, p. 19.

49. Ibid., p. 20.

50. Ibid., p. 21.

51. Ibid.

52. A. Keith Mant, "The Medical Definition of Death," pp. 218–232 in Edwin S. Schneidman, ed., *Death: Current Perspectives*, Palo Alto, Calif.: Mayfield Publishing Co. 1976, p. 227.

53. Michael Crichton, *The Great Train Robbery,* New York: Knopf, 1975, p. 73.

54. *The Times of London,* "Conference of Medical Royal Colleges Criticizes *Panorama* as Biased," November 7, 1980.

55. Richard Selzer, *Mortal Lessons: Notes on the Art of Surgery,* New York: Simon and Schuster, 1974, p. 16.

56. Brian Clark, *Whose Life Is It Anyway?,* Ashover, Derbyshire, England: Amber Lane Press, 1978.

57. Z. J. Lipowski and Anne M. Stewart, "Illness as Subjective Experience," *Psychiatry in Medicine* 4 (1973): 155–171, p. 155.

58. Chad H. Calland, "Iatrogenic Problems in End Stage Renal Failure," *New England Journal of Medicine* 287 (1973): 334–336, p. 334.

59. Michel Foucault, *The History of Sexuality: Volume 1—An Introduction,* New York: Pantheon, 1978, p. 4.

60. Calland, 1973, p. 335.

61. "Both Ends of the Stethoscope: Interview with Dr. David J. Peters," *San Diego Physician,* October, 1979: 30–37, p. 30.

62. Ibid., p. 31.

63. Irving Yalom, "Group Therapy with the Terminally Ill," paper presented at the annual meeting of the American Psychiatric Association, Miami Beach, Fla., 1976, pp. 6–7.

64. Quoted in David E. Stannard, *The Puritan Way of Death,* New York: Oxford University Press, 1977, p. 33.

65. Ariès, 1982, pp. 566–567.

66. T. R. Harrison, Paul B. Beeson, George W. Thorn, William H. Resnik, and M. M. Wintrobe, *Principles of Internal Medicine,* Philadelphia, Pa.: The Blakiston Company, 1950, p. 4.

67. Ibid.

68. Ibid.

69. Max Pinner and Benjamin F. Miller, *When Doctors Are Patients,* New York: W. W. Norton, 1952, p. xi.

70. R. Grene, *Sick Doctors,* London: Heinemann, 1971, quoted in Lipowski and Stewart, 1973, p. 155.

71. Quoted in Anne C. Roark, "Medical Educators Fear Their Schools' Curricula are Becoming Obsolete," *The Chronicle of Higher Education* 11, no. 17, November 3, 1980.

72. Balint, 1957, p. 216.

73. Joseph B. DeLee, *The Principles and Practice of Obstetrics,* 1st ed., Philadelphia, Pa.: W. B. Saunders, 1914, p. 117.

74. Alice Allgaier, "Alternative Birth Centers Offer Family Centered Care," *Hospitals* 52 (December, 1978): 97–112, p. 97.

75. Sandol Stoddard, *The Hospice Movement: A Better Way of Caring for the Dying,* Briarcliff Manor, N.Y.: Stein and Day, 1978, p. 4.

76. Ariès, 1982, p. 592.

CHAPTER FOUR

1. Michelle Harrison, *A Woman in Residence,* New York: Random House, 1982.

2. William Osler, *The Principles and Practice of Medicine,* 1st ed., New York: D. Appleton and Company, 1892, p. 1001.

3. Ibid., pp. 1001–1002.

4. Ibid., pp. 1004–1005.

5. William Osler, *The Principles and Practice of Modern Medicine,* 3rd ed., New York: D. Appleton and Company, 1899, p. 381.

6. Sir William Osler and Thomas McCrae, *The Principles and Practice of Modern Medicine,* 9th ed., New York: D. Appleton and Company, 1921, p. 388.

7. Alexander Lambert, "Alcohol," pp. 157–202 in William Osler, ed., *Modern Medicine: Its Theory and Practice,* Philadelphia: Lea Brothers, 1907, p. 158.

8. Ibid., p. 201.

9. Karl M. Vogel, "Translator's Preface," pp. 5–6 in Rudolph Schmidt, *Pain: Its·Causation and Diagnostic Significance in Internal Diseases,* 2d ed., Philadelphia: J. B. Lippincott, 1911, p. 5.

10. Schmidt, 1911, pp. 24–29.

11. Richard J. Behan, *Pain: Its Origin, Conduction, Perception and Diagnostic Significance,* New York: D. Appleton and Company, 1922, p. 13.

12. Ibid.

13. Ibid., p. 82.

14. This certainly is the image created by much of the good work done recently in medical sociology. A recent study of surgeons (Charles Bosk: *Forgive and Remember: Managing Medical Failure,* Chicago, Ill.: University of Chicago Press, 1979) is a good example. Surgeons and surgeons-in-training view their work as a "calling." They adhere to strict, demanding schedules and develop their own internal codes of conduct. They handle technical errors ritualistically and quickly, but they deal with those who transgress the moral rules of the community of surgeons pitilessly. In an appendix to his book, Bosk, explaining how he gained the

trust of his informants, tells how he acted as a conduit for news from the "outside world." Bosk increased his access to "inside" information by bringing newspapers purchased at the hospital gift stand to residents and interns on the surgical floors. Bosk says, "Their general reluctance to pick such papers up is not so much a mark of their frugality as a symbolic statement about their relationship to the world outside Pacific Hospital. I later learned that housestaff attach a magical property to newspapers, books, and magazines. If they bring them in to work they see this as jinxing themselves and condemning the group to an impossibly busy day. It is, however, permissible for outsiders to bring such taboo items to them" (p. 195).

15. Michel Foucault, *Herculine Barbin: Being the Recently Discovered Memoirs of a Nineteenth Century French Hermaphrodite,* New York: Pantheon, 1980, p. 69.

16. Ibid., p. 77.

17. Ibid.

18. Ibid., p. 78.

19. Ibid., p. 80.

20. *Oxford English Dictionary,* Oxford: Oxford University Press, 1971, p. 714.

21. Foucault, 1980, p. 131. Quote is from a paper originally published as E. Goujon, "A Study of a Case of Incomplete Hermaphroditism in a Man," *Journal de l'anatomie et de la Physiologie de l'Homme,* 1869, pp. 609–639.

22. Foucault, 1980, pp. xi, viii.

23. Ashley Montagu, *The Elephant Man: A Study in Human Dignity,* New York: E. P. Dutton, 1979, p. 13.

24. Ibid., p. 17.

25. Ibid., p. 21.

26. Ibid., p. 27.

27. Ibid., pp. 27–28.

28. Henry A. Christian, *The Principles and Practice of Modern Medicine,* 14th ed., New York: Appleton-Century, 1942, p. 2.

29. Ibid., p. 524.

30. Henry A. Christian, *The Principles and Practice of Modern Medicine,* 16th ed., New York: Appleton-Century, 1947, p. 2.

31. A. McGehee Harvey, Leighton E. Cluff, Richard J. Jones, Albert H. Owens, David Rabinowitz, and Richard S. Ross, eds., *The Principles*

*and Practice of Modern Medicine,* 17th ed., New York: Appleton-Century-Crofts, 1968, p. 1018.

32. A. McGehee Harvey, Richard J. Jones, Albert H. Owens, and Richard S. Ross, eds., *The Principles and Practice of Modern Medicine,* 18th ed., New York: Appleton-Century-Crofts, 1972, p. 1490.

33. Ibid., p. 1489.

34. Ibid., p. 1491.

35. A. McGehee Harvey, Richard J. Jones, Victor A. McKusick, Albert H. Owens, and Richard S. Ross, eds., *The Principles and Practice of Modern Medicine,* 20th ed., New York: Appleton-Century-Crofts, 1980, p. 1449.

36. Ibid., pp. 1450–1451. The section on alcoholism in Kurt Isselbacher, Raymond D. Adams, Eugene Braunwald, Robert G. Petersdorf, and Jean D. Wilson, eds., *Harrison's Principles of Internal Medicine,* 9th ed., New York: McGraw-Hill, 1980, pp. 969–977, is more explicit about the three dimensions of alcoholism. Corresponding to the physical-psychological-social problem complex is a tripartite treatment regimen. Physicians, the text says, "may be asked to help patients conquer their alcoholic tendencies or to diagnose and treat the numerous diseases to which they are subject; often they must admit or commit patients to a general or mental hospital . . . ; and lastly, they may be required to enlist the aid of available social agencies. . ." (p. 969).

37. T. R. Harrison, Paul B. Beeson, George W. Thorn, William H. Resnik, and M. M. Wintrobe, *Principles of Internal Medicine,* 1st ed., Philadelphia: The Blakiston Company, 1950.

38. Ibid., p. 9.

39. Macdonald Critchley, ed., *Butterworth's Medical Dictionary,* 2d ed., London: Butterworths, 1978.

CHAPTER FIVE

1. See Harry Braverman, *Labor and Monopoly Capital: The Degradation of Work in the Twentieth Century,* New York: Monthly Review Press, 1974, pp. 85–138 for a description of "Taylorism," as scientific management has come to be called.

2. René Dubos, *Man Adapting,* New Haven, Conn.: Yale University Press, 1965, pp. 446–448.

3. Kurt J. Isselbacher, Raymond D. Adams, Eugene Braunwald,

Robert G. Petersdorf, and Jean D. Wilson, eds., *Harrison's Principles of Internal Medicine*, 9th ed., New York: McGraw-Hill, 1980, p. 1.

4. Clifford B. Lull and Robert A. Hingson, *Control of Pain in Childbirth*, 2d ed., Philadelphia: J.B. Lippincott, 1945, pp. 114–116. See also William Ray Arney and Jane Neill, "The Location of Pain in Childbirth: Natural Childbirth and the Transformation of Obstetrics," *Sociology of Health and Illness* 4 (1982): 1–24.

5. H. Lloyd Miller, Francis E. Flannery, and Dorothy Bell, "Education for Childbirth in Private Practice: 450 Consecutive Cases," *American Journal of Obstetrics and Gynecology* 63 (1952): 792–799, p. 798.

6. René Dubos, *Man, Medicine, and Environment*, New York: Praeger, 1968, p. 64.

7. Dubos, 1965, p. xxii.

8. Ibid., p. 455.

9. N. Detounis, "On Teaching Psychosomatic Medicine to Medical Students," pp. 68–70 in *Psychosomatic Medicine in Obstetrics and Gynaecology, Third International Congress, London, 1971*, Basel: Karger, 1972, p. 68.

10. See, for example, Robert A. Hoekelman, Saul Blatman, Philip A. Brunell, Stanford B. Friedman, Henry M. Seidel, eds., *Principles of Pediatrics: Health Care of the Young*, New York: McGraw-Hill, 1978.

11. George L. Engel, "The Need for a New Medical Model: A Challenge for Biomedicine," *Science* 196 (1977): 129–136.

12. Ludwig von Bertalanffy, "An Outline of General Systems Theory," *British Journal of Philosophical Science* 1 (1950): 139–164; Ludwig von Bertalanffy, "The Theory of Open Systems in Physics and Biology," *Science* 111 (1950): 23–29; Ludwig von Bertalanffy, *General System Theory: Foundations, Development, Applications*, New York: George Braziller, 1968. See also L. von Bertalanffy, C. G. Hempel, R. E. Bass, and H. Jonas, "General System Theory: A New Approach to the Unity of Science," I–VI, *Human Biology* 23 (1951): 302–361.

13. Kenneth Walker, *The Circle of Life: A Search for an Attitude to Pain, Disease, Old Age and Death*, London: Jonathan Cape, 1942, p. 29.

14. Ibid., pp. 12–13.

15. Howard Brody, "The Systems View of Man: Implications for Medicine, Science, and Ethics," *Perspectives in Biology and Medicine* 17 (Autumn, 1973): 71–92, pp. 72–73.

16. Alan Sheldon, "Toward a General Theory of Disease and Medical Care," pp. 84–125 in Alan Sheldon, Frank Baker, and Curtis P. McLaughlin, eds., *Systems and Medical Care*, Cambridge, Mass.: The MIT Press, 1970, pp. 86, 88.

CHAPTER SIX

1. Howard Brody, "The Systems View of Man: Implications for Medicine, Science, and Ethics," *Perspectives in Biology and Medicine* 17 (1973): 71–92, pp. 76–77.

2. Alan Sheldon, "Toward a General Theory of Disease and Medical Care," pp. 84–125 in Alan Sheldon, Frank Baker, and Curtis P. McLaughlin, eds., *Systems and Medical Care*, Cambridge, Mass.: The MIT Press, 1970, p. 89.

3. H. E. Sigerist, *A History of Medicine*, New York: Oxford University Press, 1951, p. 320. Quoted in ibid., p. 85.

4. Michel Foucault, *The Birth of the Clinic: An Archeology of Medical Perception*, New York: Vintage, 1973, p. 35.

5. Ibid., p. 18.

6. Mary C. Jarrett, *Chronic Illness in New York City*, New York: Columbia University Press, 1933; George H. Bigelow and Herbert L. Lombard, *Cancer and Other Chronic Diseases in Massachusetts*, Boston: Houghton Mifflin, 1933.

7. National Health Survey, 1935–36, *The Magnitude of the Chronic Disease Problem in the United States*, Washington, D.C.: Public Health Service, 1938.

8. Joint Committee on Chronic Disease, *America's Health*, New York: Harper and Brothers, 1949.

9. Commission on the Health Needs of the Nation, *Building America's Health: A Report to the President*, Washington, D.C.: Government Printing Office, 1953.

10. Ernst P. Boas, *The Unseen Plague: Chronic Disease*, New York: J. J. Augustin Publisher, 1940, p. 5.

11. Joseph Earle Moore and David Seegal, "Announcement," *Journal of Chronic Disease* 1 (1955): 1–11, p. 2. Quote is from the Commission on the Health Needs of the Nation, 1953.

12. Ibid.

13. Ivan B. Pless and Philip Pinkerton, *Chronic Childhood Disor-*

*ders: Promoting Patterns of Adjustment,* London: Henry Kimpton, 1975, p. 21.

14. Foucault, 1973, p. 17.

15. Jurgen Ruesch, *Chronic Disease and Psychological Invalidism: A Psychosomatic Study,* New York: The American Society for Research in Psychosomatic Problems, 1946, p. 3.

16. Boas, 1940, p. 4.

17. William Osler, *The Treatment of Disease: The Address in Medicine before The Ontario Medical Association, June 7, 1909,* London: Henry Frowde, 1909, p. 6.

18. Commission of Chronic Illness, *Chronic Illness in the United States, Volume 1: Prevention of Chronic Illness,* Cambridge, Mass.: Harvard University Press, 1957, pp. xvi, 6.

19. Boas, 1940, p. 16.

20. Len Hughes, Mary O'Hara Devereaux, Ronald Singler, and Fred M. Mitchell, "The Health Care Team," pp. 128–139 in Robert B. Taylor, ed., *Family Medicine: Principles and Practice,* New York: Springer-Verlag, 1978.

21. Sheldon, 1970, p. 120.

22. Kurt J. Isselbacher, Raymond D. Adams, Eugene Braunwald, Robert G. Petersdorf, and Jean D. Wilson, eds., *Harrison's Principles of Internal Medicine,* 9th ed., New York: McGraw-Hill, 1980, p. 120.

23. Brody, 1973, p. 82.

24. Sheldon, 1970, p. 121.

25. Moore and Seegal, 1955, p. 3.

26. Dean W. Roberts, "Care of the Long-Term Patient: A Summary of the National Conference," *Journal of Chronic Disease* 1 (1955): 51–62, pp. 52, 55.

27. Moore and Seegal, 1955, p. 3.

28. Isselbacher et al., 1980, p. 9.

29. A. McGehee Harvey, Richard J. Johns, Victor A. McKusick, Albert H. Owens and Richard S. Ross, eds., *The Principles and Practice of Modern Medicine,* 20th ed., New York: Appleton-Century-Crofts, 1980, p. 12.

30. Ibid., p. 3.

31. Ibid., p. 4.

32. Ibid., p. 35.

33. Isselbacher et al., 1980, p. 2.

34. Harvey et al., 1980, p. 35.

35. Brody, 1973, p. 83.

36. Isselbacher et al., 1980, p. 10.

37. Ibid.

38. Harvey et al., 1980, p. 35.

39. Sheldon, 1970, pp. 120–121.

40. Isselbacher et al., 1980, p. 2.

41. Ibid.

42. Brody, 1973, p. 84.

43. Isselbacher et al., 1980, p. 11.

44. Brody, 1973, p. 85.

45. Ivan Illich, *Medical Nemesis: The Expropriation of Health,* New York: Pantheon, 1976.

46. Robert A. Hoekelman, Saul Blatman, Philip A. Brunell, Stanford B. Friedman, and Henry M. Seidel, eds., *Principles of Pediatrics: Health Care of the Young,* New York: McGraw-Hill, 1978, p. 16.

47. Raymond S. Duff, "On Deciding the Use of the Family Commons," *Birth Defects: Original Articles* 12 (1976): 73–84.

48. Garrett Hardin, "The Tradgedy of the Commons," *Science* 162 (1968): 1243–1248.

49. Hoekelman et al., 1978, p. 3.

50. Isselbacher et al., 1980, p. 4.

51. Hoekelman et al., 1978, p. 16.

52. Sheldon, 1970, p. 118.

53. Talcott Parsons, "Research with Human Subjects and the 'Professional Complex,' " *Daedalus* 98 (1969): 325–360, pp. 326–327, 350.

54. Harvey et al., 1980, pp. 10–11.

55. David L. Sackett, "Patients and Therapies: Getting the Two Together," *New England Journal of Medicine* 298 (1978): 278–279.

56. Harvey et al., 1980, p. 40.

57. Ibid., pp. 42–43.

58. Hoekelman et al., 1978, p. 4.

59. Charles Bosk, *Forgive and Remember: Managing Medical Failure,* Chicago, Ill.: University of Chicago Press, 1980.

60. Isselbacher et al., 1980, p. 11.

61. Boyce Rensberger, "Heat 'Pictures' of Pain Expected to Aid Sufferers, Detect Fakers," *New York Times,* October 21, 1980, p. C3.

CHAPTER SEVEN

1. Jean-Paul Sartre, *Nausea,* New York: Penguin, 1965, p. 58.
2. Ibid., p. 85.
3. Ibid., p. 59.
4. Emmanuel A. Friedman, "Primigravid Labor: A Graphicostatistical Analysis," *Obstetrics and Gynecology* 6 (1955): 567–589.
5. Philip J. Steer, "Monitoring in Labor," *British Journal of Hospital Practice* 17 (1977): 219–225.
6. Elisabeth Kübler-Ross, *On Death and Dying,* New York: Macmillan, 1969.
7. Barney Glaser and Anselm Strauss, *Time for Dying,* Chicago: Aldine, 1968.
8. Raymond A. Moody, Jr., *Life after Life: The Investigation of a Phenomenon—Survival of Bodily Death,* Atlanta: Mockingbird Books, 1975.
9. A. McGehee Harvey, Richard J. Johns, Victor A. McKusick, Albert H. Owens, and Richard S. Ross, eds., *The Principles and Practice of Modern Medicine,* 20th ed., New York: Appleton-Century-Crofts, 1980, p. 44.
10. Kenneth Ring, *Life at Death: A Scientific Investigation of the Near Death Experience,* New York: Coward, McCann and Geohegan, 1980.
11. Richard A. Kalish, ed., *Death, Dying, Transcending,* Farmingdale, N.Y.: Baywood Publishing Co., 1980, p. 2.
12. Ring, 1980, p. 263.
13. Richard A. Kalish, ed., *Caring Relationships: The Dying and the Bereaved,* Farmingdale, NY: Baywood Publishing Co., 1980, p. 7.
14. Jacob Swartz and Paul Kaufman, "Medical Care and the Emotional Life of the Patient," pp. 8–29 in Robert L. Wilkins and Norman G. Levinsky, eds., *Medicine: Essentials of Clinical Practice,* 2d ed., Boston: Little, Brown and Company, 1978, p. 9.
15. Matilda White Riley, "Introduction: Life Course Perspectives," pp. 3–13 in Matilda White Riley, ed., *Aging from Birth to Death: Interdisciplinary Perspectives,* Boulder, Colo.: Westview Press, 1979, pp. 3–5.

16. Jacques Donzelot, *The Policing of Families,* New York: Pantheon, 1979, p. 170.

17. Joseph Earle Moore and David Seegal, "Announcement," *Journal of Chronic Disease* 1 (1955): 1–12, p. 4.

18. Commission on Chronic Illness, *Chronic Illness in the United States, Volume 1: Prevention of Chronic Illness,* Cambridge, Mass.: Harvard University Press, 1957, p. 120.

19. Dean W. Roberts, "Care of the Long-Term Patient: A Summary of the National Conference," *Journal of Chronic Disease* 1 (1955): 51–62, pp. 54, 57, 58.

20. Commission on Chronic Illness, 1957, p. 4.

21. Moore and Seegal, 1955, pp. 4–5.

22. Michel Foucault, "Introduction," pp. ix-xx in Georges Canguilhem, *On the Normal and the Pathological,* Boston: D. Reidel Publishing, 1978, p. xix.

23. Commission on Chronic Illness, 1957, p. xv.

24. Ernst P. Boas, *The Unseen Plague: Chronic Disese,* New York: J. J. Augustin Publisher, 1940, p. 14.

25. Moore and Seegal, 1955, p. 2.

26. R. J. Haggerty, "Foreword," pp. 11–12 in Ivan B. Pless and Philip Pinkerton, *Chronic Childhood Disorders: Promoting Patterns of Adjustment,* London: Henry Kimpton, 1975, p. 12.

27. Grantly Dick-Read, *Childbirth without Fear,* London: Heinemann, 1933.

28. Hillary Graham, "Images of Pregnancy in Antenatal Literature," pp. 15–37 in Robert Dingwall, Christian Heath, Margaret Reid, and Margaret Stacey, eds., *Health Care and Health Knowledge,* London: Croom Helm, 1977.

29. Sheila Kitzinger, *The Experience of Childbirth,* London: Victor Gollancz, 1962; Sheila Kitzinger, *Education and Counselling for Childbirth,* London: Ballière Tindall, 1977; Sheila Kitzinger, *Giving Birth: The Parents' Emotions in Childbirth,* New York: Schocken, 1977.

30. Sheila Kitzinger, "The Woman on the Delivery Table," pp. 91–111 in Margaret Irene Laing, ed., *Woman on Woman,* London: Sedgwick and Jackson, 1971, p. 93.

31. Kitzinger, 1971, p. 105. See also Susan G. Doering and Doris R. Entwisle, "Preparation during Pregnancy and Ability to Cope with Labor

and Delivery," *American Journal of Orthopsychiatry* 45 (1975): 825–837, p. 835.

32. Herbert Thoms and Robert H. Wyatt, "One Thousand Consecutive Deliveries under a Training for Childbirth Program," *American Journal of Obstetrics and Gynecology* 61 (1951): 205–209, p. 206.

33. Carl Tupper, "Conditioning for Childbirth," *American Journal of Obstetrics and Gynecology* 71 (1956): 733–740, p. 739.

34. Ibid., p. 735.

35. Lyn H. Lofland, *The Craft of Dying: The Modern Face of Death,* Beverly Hills, Calif.: Sage, 1978, pp. 75–76.

36. David Cole Gordon, *Overcoming the Fear of Death,* New York: Macmillan, 1970, p. 108, quoted in Lofland, 1978, p. 99.

37. Susan G. Doering, Doris R. Entwisle, and Daniel Quinlan, "Modeling the Quality of Women's Birth Experience," *Journal of Health and Social Behavior* 21 (1980): 12–21, p. 13, italics added.

38. Lofland, 1978, pp. 99, 100.

39. Ibid., p. 79.

40. Robert J. Kastenbaum, "Introduction: Toward Standards of Care for the Terminally Ill," pp. 1–6 in Kalish, *Caring Relationships,* 1980, pp. 4–5.

41. Richard C. Erikson and Bobbie J. Hyerstay, "The Dying Patient and the Double Bind Hypothesis," pp. 18–29 in Kalish, *Death, Dying, Transcending,* 1980, pp. 26, 27.

42. Harold M. Schmeck, Jr., "Life-Span Research Predicts Healthier, but Not Longer, Old Age," *New York Times,* October 21, 1980, pp. C1, C3.

43. Harvey et al., 1980, p. 15.

44. Swartz and Kaufman, 1978, p. 13.

45. Robert L. Kahn, "Aging and Social Support," pp. 77–91 in Riley, 1979, p. 85.

46. Paul B. Baltes and Sherry L. Willis, "Life-Span Developmental Psychology, Cognitive Functioning, and Social Policy," pp. 15–46 in Riley, 1979, p. 34.

47. Swartz and Kaufman, 1978, p. 8.

48. Robert A. Hoekelman, Saul Blatman, Philip A. Brunnell, Stanford B. Friedman, and Henry M. Seidel, eds., *Principles of Pediatrics: Health Care of the Young,* New York: McGraw-Hill, 1978, p. 6.

49. Sidney Cobb, "Social Support and Health Throughout the Life Course," pp. 93–106 in Riley, 1979, p. 103.

50. Ibid.

51. Ivan Illich, *Medical Nemesis: The Expropriation of Health*, New York: Bantam, 1976, p. 202.

CHAPTER EIGHT

1. Carlo M. Cipolla, *Faith, Reason, and the Plague in Seventeenth-Century Tuscany*, Ithaca, N.Y.: Cornell University Press, 1979.

2. Ibid., pp. 8, 7.

3. William Ryan, *Blaming the Victim*, New York: Vintage Books, 1976, p. 7.

4. Ibid., p. 25.

5. Ibid., p. 29.

6. Barry Blackwell, "Patient Compliance," *New England Journal of Medicine* 289 (1973): 249–252, p. 250.

7. Ibid., p. 252.

8. Marc Renaud, "On the Structural Constraints to State Intervention in Health," *International Journal of Health Services* 5 (1975): 559–571, p. 567. Renaud was speaking of the HEW report, *Work in America: Report of a Special Task Force to the Secretary of Health, Education, and Welfare*, Cambridge, Mass.: The MIT Press, 1973.

9. Jane E. Brody, "Study Suggests Changing Behavior May Prevent Heart Attack," *New York Times*, September 16, 1980, pp. C1, C3.

10. Ivan Illich, *Medical Nemesis: The Expropriation of Health*, New York: Bantam Books, 1976.

11. Rick Carlson, *The End of Medicine*, New York: John Wiley and Sons, 1975.

12. Victor R. Fuchs, *Who Shall Live? Health, Economics, and Social Choice*, New York: Basic Books, 1974.

13. Ibid., pp. 4–5.

14. Ibid., p. 149.

15. Ibid., p. 151.

16. Howard S. Berliner, "Emerging Ideologies in Medicine," *Review of Radical Political Economics* 9, no. 1 (1977): 116–123, p. 119.

17. John Knowles, *Conference on Future Directions in Health Care: The Dimensions of Medicine*. Sponsored by Blue Cross Association, The Rockefeller Foundation, and Health Policy Program, University of Cali-

fornia, New York, December, 1975, pp. 2, 3. Quoted in Robert Crawford, "You are Dangerous to Your Health: The Ideology and Politics of Victim Blaming," *International Journal of Health Services* 7 (1977): 663–680, p. 663.

18. Walter McNerney, *Conference on Future Directions in Health Care*, p. 5, quoted in Crawford, 1977, p. 664.

19. Cipolla, 1979, pp. 87–92. See also Carlo M. Cipolla, *Cristofano and the Plague*, Berkeley, Calif.: University of California Press, 1973.

20. Michel Foucault, *Discipline and Punish: The Birth of the Prison*, London: Allen Lane, 1977, p. 198.

21. Ibid., p. 194.

22. Eleanor Lake, "Trouble on the Street Corners," *Reader's Digest* 42 (May, 1943): 43–46, from *Common Sense*, May, 1943, p. 43.

23. Ibid.

24. Quoted in ibid., p. 44.

25. Quoted in Gladys Denny Schultz, "Does Your Daughter Think She's in Love?" *Reader's Digest* 44 (May, 1944): 63–64, from *Better Homes and Gardens*, March, 1944, p. 63.

26. Lake, 1943, p. 45.

27. "Must We Change Our Sex Standards?" *Reader's Digest* 52 (June, 1948): 1–6, p. 6.

28. Howard Whitman, "Let's Help Them Marry Young," *Reader's Digest* 51 (October, 1947): 1–4, from *Better Homes and Gardens*, August, 1947, p. 3.

29. Jonathan Rinehart, "Mothers without Joy," *Reader's Digest* 83 (July, 1963): 83–87, from *The Saturday Evening Post*, 23 March, 1963, pp. 83, 85.

30. Lake, 1943, p. 46.

31. Whitman, 1947, p. 1.

32. Rinehart, 1963, p. 87.

33. Alex Poinsett, "A Despised Minority," *Ebony* 21 (August, 1966): 48–55.

34. Thaddeus J. Trenn, "Ludwik Fleck's 'On the Question of the Foundations of Medical Knowledge,'" *Journal of Medicine and Philosophy* 6 (1981): 237–256, p. 245. Also see Hilary Graham, "Images of Pregnancy in Antenatal Literature," pp. 15–37 in Robert Dingwall, Christian Heath, Margaret Reid, and Margaret Stacey, eds., *Health Care and Health Knowledge*, London: Croom Helm, 1977, for an excellent study

using pictures as ideograms and for bibliographic references justifying the technique.

35. Michel Foucault, *The History of Sexuality, Volume 1—An Introduction*, New York: Pantheon, 1979.

36. Michel Foucault, ed., *Herculine Barbin: Being the Recently Discovered Memoirs of a Nineteenth Century French Hermaphrodite*, New York: Pantheon, 1981.

37. Richard Woodbury, "Help for High School Mothers," *Life* (2 April, 1971): 38–43.

38. "Must We Change Our Sex Standards? A Readers' Symposium," *Reader's Digest* 53 (September, 1948): 129–132, p. 129.

39. Ibid., p. 130.

40. James Lincoln Collier, "Sex Education—Blunt Answers for Tough Questions: An Interview with Lester A. Kirkendall," *Reader's Digest* 92 (June, 1968):80–84, p. 84.

41. The Alan Guttmacher Institute, *Teenage Pregnancy: The Problem That Hasn't Gone Away*, New York: The Alan Guttmacher Institute, 1981.

42. James Daniel, "The Case of the Pregnant Schoolgirl," *Reader's Digest* 97 (September, 1970): 169–173, from *The PTA Magazine*, June, 1970, p. 170.

43. Edwin Kiester, Jr., "The Bitter Lessons: Too Many of Our Schools Are Teaching Pregnant Teenagers," *Today's Health* 50 (June, 1972): 54–60, p. 54.

44. Kathleen Fury, "The Troubling Truth about Teenagers and Sex," *Reader's Digest* 116 (June, 1980): 153–156, from *Ladies' Home Journal*, March, 1980, p. 155.

45. Pearila Brickner Rothenberg and Phyllis E. Varga, "The Relationship between Age of Mother and Child Health and Development," *American Journal of Public Health* 71 (August, 1981): 810–815.

46. Naomi M. Morris, "The Biological Advantages and Social Disadvantages of Teenage Pregnancy," *American Journal of Public Health* 71 (August, 1981): 796, p. 796.

47. Ibid.

48. Daniel, 1970, pp. 170–171.

49. Kiester, 1972, p. 60.

50. Ted Rosenthal, *How Could I Not Be Among You?* New York: Avon, 1973, p. 29.

51. Ibid., pp. 26–27.

52. Ibid., p. 73.

CHAPTER NINE
1. John F. Burnam, "Sounding Board: The Physician as a Double Agent," *New England Journal of Medicine* 297 (1977): 278–279, p. 278.
2. Ibid.
3. Robert F. Murray, "The Practitioner's View of the Values Involved in Genetic Screening and Counseling: Individual vs. Societal Imperatives," pp. 185–199 in Daniel Bergsma, ed., *Ethical, Social, and Legal Dimensions of Screening for Human Genetic Disease*, New York: Stratton, 1974, p. 198.
4. Burnam, 1977, p. 279.
5. Jeffrey Lionel Berlant, *Profession and Monopoly: A Study of Medicine in the United States and Great Britain*, Berkeley, Calif.: University of California Press, 1975, p. 115.
6. Ibid., p. 118.
7. Daniel Callahan, "To Confront Ethical Issues in Medicine," *New England Journal of Medicine* 292 (1975): 315–316, p. 315.
8. Raymond S. Duff and A. G. M. Campbell, "Moral and Ethical Dilemmas in the Special Care Nursery," *New England Journal of Medicine* 289 (1973): 890–894.
9. Anthony Shaw, "Dilemmas of 'Informed Consent' in Children," *New England Journal of Medicine* 289 (1973): 885–890.
10. Callahan, 1975, p. 315.
11. Ibid.
12. Stephen E. Toulmin, *An Examination of the Place of Reason in Ethics*, Cambridge: Cambridge University Press, 1950, p. 202.
13. K. Danner Clouser, "Medical Ethics: Some Uses, Abuses, and Limitations," *New England Journal of Medicine* 293 (1975): 384–387, p. 387.
14. Talcott Parsons, "Research with Human Subjects and the 'Profession Complex,' " *Daedalus* 98 (1969): 325–360, p. 327.
15. Eric J. Cassell, "Autonomy and Ethics in Action," *New England Journal of Medicine* 297 (1977): 333–334, p. 334.
16. Ibid., pp. 333, 334.
17. Robert A. Hoekelman, Saul Blatman, Philip A. Brunell, Stanford B. Friedman, and Henry M. Seidel, eds., *Principles of Pediatrics: Health Care of the Young*, New York: McGraw-Hill, 1978, pp. 6–7.
18. Clouser, 1975, p. 387.

19. Ibid., p. 385.

20. John Lachs, "Humane Care and the Treatment of Humans," *New England Journal of Medicine* 294 (1976): 838–840, p. 839, italics added.

21. Joseph Fletcher, "Indicators of Humanhood: A Tentative Profile of Man," *The Hastings Center Report* 2 (1972): 1–4, p. 4.

22. Kenneth E. Boulding, "Sociobiology or Biosociology?," *Society* 15, no. 6, (1978): 28–34.

23. Edward O. Wilson, *Sociobiology: The New Synthesis*, Cambridge, Mass.: Harvard University Press, 1975.

24. Edward O. Wilson, "Introduction: What is Sociobiology?," pp. 1–12 in Michael S. Gregory, Anita Silvers, and Diane Sutch, eds., *Sociobiology and Human Nature*, San Francisco: Jossey-Bass, 1978, p. 2.

25. Lionel Tiger, *Optimism: The Biology of Hope*, New York: Simon and Schuster, 1979, p. 22.

26. Wilson, 1978, pp. 7–8.

27. Tiger, 1979, p. 15.

28. Ibid., p. 21.

29. George Edin Pugh, *The Biological Origin of Human Values*, New York: Basic Books, 1977, pp. 5, 11.

30. John L. Fuller, "Genes, Brains, and Behavior," pp. 98–115 in Gregory et al., 1978, p. 99.

31. J. B. Schneewind, "Sociobiology, Social Policy, and Nirvana," pp. 225–239 in Gregory et al., 1978, p. 226.

32. Henry E. Kelly, "Biosociology and Crime," pp. 87–99 in C. R. Jeffery, ed., *Biology and Crime*, Beverly Hills, Calif.: Sage Publications, 1979, p. 90.

33. Kelly, pp. 98–99.

34. Wilson, 1978, p. 4.

35. Kai T. Erikson, *Everything in Its Path: Destruction of Community in the Buffalo Creek Flood*, New York: Simon and Schuster, 1976, pp. 193–194.

36. Schneewind, 1978, pp. 231–232.

37. Hoekelman et al., 1978, pp. 4, 5, 6.

38. See Marshall H. Klaus and John H. Kennell, *Maternal-Infant Bonding: The Impact of Early Separation or Loss on Family Development*, St. Louis, Mo.: Mosby, 1976. Their original paper on bonding appeared as M. H. Klaus, R. Jerauld, N. C. Kreger, W. McAlpine, M. Steffa, and

J. H. Kennell, "Maternal Attachment: Importance of the First Post-Partum Days," *New England Journal of Medicine* 286 (1972): 460–463.

39. William Ray Arney, "Maternal-Infant Bonding: The Politics of Falling in Love with Your Child," *Feminist Studies* 6 (1980): 547–570, reviews the literature on the effects of not being bonded.

40. Roberto Sousa, John Kennell, Marshall Klaus, Steven Robertson, and Juan Urrutia, "The Effect of a Supportive Companion on Perinatal Problems, Length of Labor, and Mother Infant Interaction," *New England Journal of Medicine* 303 (1980): 597–600.

41. Kenneth Ring, *Life at Death: A Scientific Investigation of the Near-Death Experience,* New York: Coward, McCann, and Geohegan, 1980, pp. 15, 216–217.

42. Ibid., p. 251.

43. Ibid., p. 255.

44. In an early essay Michel Foucault connects the emergence of a modern language of sexuality directly to the disappearance of a language of spirituality. The search for sexuality has replaced the search for God as the means for approaching the limits of being, Foucault argues. Thus, it is not surprising to see the language of sexuality seep into the spaces around medicine left by the excision of spirituality. See Michel Foucault, "A Preface to Transgression," pp. 29–52 in Donald F. Bouchard, ed., *Language, Counter-Memory, Practice: Selected Essays and Interviews by Michel Foucault,* Ithaca, N.Y.: Cornell University Press, 1977.

CHAPTER TEN

1. Michel Foucault, *The History of Sexuality, Volume 1—An Introduction,* New York: Pantheon, 1978, Chapter 1.

2. Dan Hulbert, "For Parents, Race to Harvard Starts in Nursery School," *New York Times,* January 4, 1981: EDUC 1 & EDUC 19, p. EDUC 1.

3. Graham Greene, *The Ministry of Fear: An Entertainment,* New York: Viking Press, 1943, p. 222.

4. Alfred North Whitehead, *Science and the Modern World,* quoted without reference in John P. Sisk, "The Tyranny of Harmony," *The American Scholar* 46 (1977): 193–205, p. 199.

5. Sisk, 1977.

6. Ibid., p. 205.

# Index